Light in the Closet

Biblical Insights for the M2F Transgender Journey

By Klein

AF719499

Light in the Closet
TRANSGENDER SUPPORT

For Jennifer who supported me with the love and grace that makes honest exploration possible.

lightinthecloset.org

Second paperback edition, September 2026

ISBN 978-0-9700549-9-9

Published by Klein Graphics Publishing

kleingraphicsLLC.com

The references available throughout this book are there for your convenience. Light in the Closet does not necessarily endorse all subject matter, nor can Light in the Closet vouch for the validity of content provided by third parties or obtained on the internet. Any recommendation or citation by Light in the Closet of published print, or online media is not necessarily an endorsement of any or all matter contained in that publication.

Table of Contents

Introduction

There are an estimated six million* people in the U.S. who explore gender expressions opposite their legal birth gender. Over one and a half million** of these people identify as transgender. They may feel trapped in a life that does not fit. Some, out of obligations to family, friends and career, attempt to deny or conceal these feelings. These individuals may end up living a secret, closeted life. Due to their discomfort, many deal with misplaced fear, guilt and shame.

The ministry Light in the Closet offers a safe place for individuals to research, with confidentiality, personal issues, desires and fears they are dealing with. This publication focuses on issues important to Christians and those who are seeking spiritual and emotional guidance.

This book deals in part with the topic of sin from the biblical perspective of Jesus. The teachings of Jesus revolve around the fruits of the Spirit. You can identify those who follow Jesus by the evidence of those fruits in their actions and lives. Those fruits are: peace, patience, kindness, joy, goodness, faithfulness, gentleness, self-control, and, most importantly, love. To understand the teachings in the Bible, a reader must first agree with the premise of a loving God. It is with that understanding that Light in the Closet presents these insights and articles.

---

*The figure of 6 million (who question gender identity) is out of the 13.68 million (see Clinical and Sociological Information on LITC website / 2000 Census) identified as transgender by the Human Rights Campaign (HRC) and confirmed by various groups including the American Medical Association (AMA). This figure attempts to include all individuals falling under the general category of transgender. Even so, over 95% of these are cross dressers, most of whom are closeted. Figures are estimates and due to the nature of the subject matter, hard data is difficult to gather.

**The amount of individuals who identify as transgender and living full time outwardly in their modified gender is 1.6 million in 2020. This is taken from research conducted between 2014 and 2020 by the University of California Los Angeles. There is also a very comprehensive study released in 2022 from "U.S. Transgender Survey" (see the resource section on the LITC website).

Although primarily focused on those who identify as Christian, this publication benefits anyone seeking biblical guidance concerning transgender issues. A trans person may find this information helpful if they need to effectively address concerns and accusations aimed at them.

The founder of Light in the Closet has spent decades exploring the issue of gender and how that relates to biblical teachings. We hope to encourage an honest exploration of gender identity and life-style choices.

The information and help offered is not a replacement for professional care. Those who need professional medical, clinical or psychological help should pursue those avenues.

Some may wonder if this topic is outside the scope of traditional church care. I would say that Jesus desires us to be honest with him and each other, and sometimes that honesty is a bit messy. Authenticity, honesty and vulnerability are necessary if your intention is to pursue the truth of who you are.

We can hide from ourselves so well that we do not even know we are hiding in a "closet." Closets may feel safe, but they are never places of growth. Even if you want to stay in your closet, you should allow some light in. This publication hopes to do just that so you may experience some peace, growth, and joy as you discover more about who you are in the light. Your trials and tests should not be feared but embraced as opportunities for clarity and wisdom.

> *"Even though I walk through the valley of the shadow of death, I will fear no evil, for you are with me; your rod and your staff, they comfort me." Psalm 23:3-5*[1]

Although we prefer to avoid the valleys in our lives, most valleys we must walk through. Because Jesus promises to walk through the valley with us, that journey need not be full of frustration, but an honest exploration that will lead to godly growth.

Light in the Closet - Biblical Insights for the M2F Transgender Journey was produced to show M2F (male to female) transgender individuals that Jesus will walk with them through their valley.

1 Most scripture references throughout this book are from the New American Standard Bible (NASB), © 1960, 1962, 1968, 1971, 1973, 1975, 1977, 1995 by The Lockman Foundation

Gender Identity

About Gender Identity

Gender identity is a significant part of our self-identity and how we relate to others. We see the world though the filter of our gender. Although some achievements towards a more gender-fluid society have been made, our Western culture remains gender-polarized. We treat males and females very differently. Society allows or encourages certain activities and desires for one gender and disallows them for the other gender. Most people are conditioned to accept these restrictions as they grow and develop as either men or women. They see their gender as a given and expend little energy or conscious thought on it. When they think of themselves, they are simply "Sally" or "Ted" and identify as an individual. Their gender is secondary to that. They are comfortable with their assigned gender as it relates to their identity, and are just simply male or female.

However, those with Gender Identity Disorder (GID) are always aware of their gender. They relate most of their actions as in line with one gender or the other. This preoccupation with gender will often color their choices in activities or career. They purpose to engage in only those activities they feel match their gender. These people are constantly questioning their gender and so also their identity. A trans person rejects the gender identity assigned at birth (in large part) and the social restrictions that come with it. They find themselves being herded into one gender group while desiring to be associated with the other. Their sense of self is never fully affirmed because their gender is constantly being questioned.

Without a firm sense-of-self, it is difficult to relate to others or even God.

For the transgender individual, the development of personhood beyond gender is the key to self-acceptance, social acceptance and personal growth. Befriending who you are now is important, even if you want to move ahead into something new.

About Gender Identity Disorder (GID)

Gender identity disorder (GID) and transsexualism are defined by strong, persistent feelings of identification with the opposite gender and discomfort with one's own assigned gender. People with GID desire to live as members of the opposite gender and often dress and use mannerisms associated with the other gender. For instance, a person identified as a boy may feel and act like a girl. The causes of this condition are varied but the discomfort with one's perceived gender can be equally as real in all instances. The three main causes are:

1. **Those born with ambiguous genitalia, or those who are inter-sexed (hermaphrodites).**

   This is by far the largest group diagnosed with GID. The natural processes of gender evolution in the womb that determines male and female traits proceeds with little regard to cultural acceptance.

2. **Those that have brain development skewed from their genitalia development.**

   We all start off in the womb with feminine traits. A few weeks into fetal development sexual differentiation occurs and we become distinctly male or female. However, some fetuses develop both sets of organs or have neither well defined. The end result to this physical development of the genitalia is what's known as the birth gender.

   Female and male brains are different. The determination of whether a fetus develops a typically female or male brain is influenced by a combination of factors. These are separate from those factors influencing the fetus' physiological biology. The brain can develop a distinctively different "gender" from what is evidenced by the genitalia.

   This process is natural and usually without health risks. Even so, society's rigid gender models may cause a person who demonstrates a physical and psychological gender incongruity to develop gender identity disorder.

3. **Those who have suffered emotional or physical trauma.**

   Although this is listed here as a reason for GID, the medical community does not recognize trauma or abuse as a cause for GID. GID is seen mainly as a prenatal condition. However, personal or social trauma, especially related to gender can be causes for cross-dressing (which relates mostly to fetish behavior). Most diagnoses of GID focuses on how a person feels and acts. There is no conclusive medical test or evidence for a GID diagnosis. Diagnosis of GID is often determined by observation and an individual's declaration that they are gender-incongruent. As a result, trauma as a cause for cross-dressing is sometimes diagnosed and treated as gender identity disorder.

The medical community views GID as a medical condition that needs to be fixed. Treatment for this condition includes psychological counseling, hormones, and for some, sexual reassignment surgery (SRS). This diagnosis is based on a strict adherence to the polarized gender model of male and female. Those who seek SRS feel they will be more comfortable in their new bodies and wish society to relate to them in the gender they have embraced. Some view this desire to be the "opposite" gender as a rejection of societal norms. The process of SRS actually embraces the polarized gender by rejecting one gender and conforming to the other.

The polarized gender model is what most of us in the western world understand as gender. But in the past few years this has started to change. One such model advocates for four genders: masculine, feminine, neuter, and common. Other gender models include seven, eleven and even fifty-two different gender categories. Recently proposed gender models attempt to reflect a social concept of gender as a "spectrum." We apparently have a strong need to label someone. Perhaps that is the real issue. Light in the Closet ministry recommends focusing on personhood over gender. This celebrates a person's dignity and promotes diversity.

Although research has been going on for some time regarding GID[2], good research is fairly recent and incomplete. The subject of a person's gender, and how that gender impacts a person's role in society, is open to much debate. No emphatic statement declaring absolutes should be given much consideration.

Our society is evolving and changing and how we relate to it through our gender identity is in flux as well. Some feel that the words, "gender identity"

---

2 For more information about GID you can log on at: http://www.webmd.com/sex/gender-identity-disorder

should not be linked to the word "disorder." They would advocate that to view a psychological, sociological or physical gender inconsistency as a "disorder" is a mistake of the highest order. Many feel that they do not need to be "fixed" at all, but instead have focused their energies on promoting change in our society to gain social and self-acceptance. A better term for those choosing to pursue a gender expression different from what they begin with is, "gender-congruency." Gender congruency is defined as a harmonious balance of biological gender and psychological gender identity.

Many consider themselves to be gender-fluid or bi-gender. This would be a person who's gender expression is a mix or in flux. Other gender labels which have been gaining acceptance are:*

Agender: Described as being gender neutral or genderless.

Gender queer: Used by people who do not identify with being a man or a woman, or a gender non-conforming or non-binary person.

Intersex: A person born with a reproductive or sexual anatomy that doesn't seem to fit the typical definitions of female or male. This term has been around forever.

Gender Variant: Someone who does not conform to gender-based expectations of society

Third Gender: This gender category is used by societies that recognize three or more genders and is also a conceptual term.

Two-Spirit: Used by Native American people to recognize individuals who possess qualities of both genders. Coined in 1990, Two-Spirit is a modern, pan-Indigenous umbrella term specific to North American Native cultures, but similar third-gender and gender-diverse roles exist in many different cultures globally.

No one has all the answers, and it is only through an open and honest dialogue that some relevant truths will be reached. It is for this reason that Light in the Closet supports an individual's right to prayerfully choose whichever path they follow.

*Not a complete list

Gender Euphoria

The intense "high" experienced when an individual cross-dresses (especially the first few times) is known as gender euphoria. This "high" may be experienced each time a person dresses as the "opposite" gender (to their perceived birth gender). It may take months, or even years for gender euphoria to diminish. Even for those who have cross-dressed in part for years, gender euphoria can still be experienced during that first exploration of full-enfemme. This elation is further intensified if the person is going through andropause, menopause or a change of life. A person who is chronically depressed or suffering from stress will often find a break from those negative feelings and by contrast experience even more of a rush.

The act of cross-dressing may cause the brain to release endorphins. The intensity of this high may diminish over time, and the individual may seek additional stimulation by going out more in public, taking risks, or by prolonging the cross-dressing experience. Sometimes a person may feel that this is "who they really are" inside and desire to continue in the opposite gender role full-time. This is one of many reasons why someone who is considering a radical life style change should seek out a counselor or therapist. For some, gender euphoria is one step in the process of transition. For others, gender euphoria is nothing more than an intense experience and the desire to cross-dress will diminish when the euphoria wears thin.

Endorphins are a group of substances formed within the body that naturally relieve pain. They have a similar chemical structure to morphine. In addition to their analgesic and pain-relieving effects, endorphins are thought to be involved in controlling the body's response to stress, determining mood. They may also regulate the release of hormones from the pituitary gland, notably growth hormone and the gonadotropin hormones.

It is common knowledge that exercise can release endorphins into the blood stream. Endorphins are also released during orgasm, simple laughter and during the act of cross-dressing. Activities that release endorphins may help to relieve stress and depression. The act of cross-dressing may actually help treat depression and could be used as a form of self-prescribed therapy. A Duke University study released in 2000 showed that, for some people, a routine of exercising was as effective in lessening depression as taking the antidepressant Zoloft.

Cross-dressing itself will not lead to depression, but the potential guilt associated with it can. Depression however, may lead to cross-dressing in order to get relief from the depression. Like anything else, cross-dressing can be abused. People can get addicted to cross-dressing because of the endorphin high they get and during this high get a break from their other problems.

If your life is in order and you are using cross-dressing for an occasional release of tension, then you may not have a problem. However, if your cross-dressing is isolating you and you are feeling anxious, frustrated or lonely then you may want to seek out a professional therapist you can talk with. There is a difference between avoiding problems in your life and finding ways to relax while you deal with them.

In the end, it's up to you to figure out whether or not cross-dressing is fitting into your life in a positive way. If it isn't, the next step is to figure out why. The articles and resources in this publication may help. If you seek out a counselor to help work through your concerns, be sure they are knowledgeable about gender issues, and have more than one client.

11 Common Questions From a Spouse of an M2F

It is still difficult to find good solid support systems for the spouses of those who are closeted. Often, when the wife discovers their husband is a closeted cross-dresser, she finds herself in the closet as well. Information and help may be hard to find, but not impossible. She will have many questions.

Here are 11 common questions along with some short answers. I hope these help.

1. **Is my husband gay?**

A: Usually not. Most men who cross-dress are straight. The percentage of men who cross-dress and are gay is no different then the percentage of gay men in the general population. Perhaps 10% or less. There is a difference between gender identity and sexual orientation, and the issue of cross-dressing has to do with gender identity.

2. **Is it my fault?**

A: It is very unlikely that the wife is ever the cause of a husband's cross-dressing. Usually this has to do with gender identity, and is something they were prone to well before you ever met him.

3. **Are the children in psychological danger?**

A: Usually cross-dressing in secret has little or no impact on the children. Even if they know or suspect something, most children are focused in on their own needs and wants. If these are being met and the child feels loved, then the relationship normally is unaffected. It is best to talk with the children in an open and age specific manner. There is a long article under "Should I Tell?" titled, "How to Begin a Conversation With Your Children." (see page 122)

4. **Are the children in physical danger?**

A: Not from the act of cross-dressing. In fact, those who are male with a gender identity disorder and are able to express themselves as female, are often less frustrated and easier to get along with than those who are suppressing these feelings. If you do suspect physical abuse, this is a separate issue and should be dealt with regardless of your husband's other issues.

5. **Is this just a phase?**

A: For those with gender identity disorder, that condition is one that more than likely existed since the womb. His thinking patterns and gender expressions are ingrained in him and really cannot change. However, how he handles these thoughts and feelings may change. The expression of cross-dressing itself may be just a phase, especially if the reason behind the cross-dressing has to do with some issue your husband is working out. Perhaps he is trying to come to grips with past abuse? If this is the case, then this phase may be important for him in regards to therapy. Either way, it is best to focus in on the cause or reason behind the cross-dressing and not the cross-dressing itself. A trained therapist can help with this process.

6. **I thought I had married a strong man. Why is he so weak?**

A: If your husband is dealing with a gender identity issue and is over the age of 30, then I would say he is a strong person indeed. Since this group is so heavily closeted it is difficult to get good information, however, it is a known fact that nearly half of those who identify as transgender attempt suicide before the age of 20. Over 50% of those who are transgender die by the age of 30. If this is any indication of what your husband has struggled with and he is still around, then I would say that he is strong indeed.

7. **How will others look at me and the children if they know my husband is a cross-dresser?**

A: The first question a person asks when they find out that a married man is a cross-dresser is, "How does your wife feel about this?" Followed closely by... "Do your children know?" Most relatives and friends of the family are more interested on how this impacts the man's family than any personal question they might have for the husband and/or father. Usually the reaction the wife gets from others is sympathy. It is also up to her to set-the-tone for the acceptance or the rejection of the husband by friends, church congregation, co-workers and family. If she is vocally negative, the response by-and-large from others will be negative as well. If she is supportive or at least understanding, then acceptance by others is much higher. The wife sets the tone for future interaction. If she demonstrates that this is a private matter, then the issue will usually remain so.

8. **I thought we had good marriage. Is it over now?**

A: If you have had a good marriage before you knew he was a cross-dresser, then your marriage should be able to stand up to this latest challenge. In fact, his keeping this information to himself was a wall between you both and now that wall has come down. It may not seem so now, but you have the opportunity to partner with him and the two of you could even grow closer as a result. If your marriage was bad before, then this could become a lightning rod for all the hurt you have felt and an excuse to end the relationship. Those who take their vows seriously to love each other find this can be a time of healing and closeness. If you can find a way to accept him, chances are he will never leave you and love you all the more.

9. **I am in over my head. What am I going to do?**

A: Yes, you are in over your head. If this is all new to you, you should know that the learning curve is steep. There are many things you can or should do. Here are a few in order:

First of all, allow yourself the freedom to cry or yell. What you are feeling is normal and your response healthy.

Second, give yourself time to process this information. He has upset the apple cart of your marriage and it will take time to clean up this mess. Hopefully he came out to you looking for support, but even if you have found out this information on your own (which is harder on you), he still needs your support. If he has been unfaithful as well, then you both need support and a marriage counselor should be a top priority.

Third, seek out help or someone to talk with. You may feel as if your world has flipped right now, and are unsure what to do with this information. Although you may not know where to turn, it is important to find someone you can bounce your feelings off of. This is primarily your husband's issue, but he has made it yours as well. If your church has a Stephen Minister you can talk with, that could be a good resource. Anyone that you know who will keep a confidence might be another option. Your "best friend" might not automatically be the best choice. Going to your head pastor, your husband's boss, his mother or a family member may only make things worse. Seek out someone, perhaps a professional therapist who understands gender identity, who is not directly connected to your community.

Fourth, connect with your husband and let him know you love him. This is a great opportunity to show the compassion and love of Christ. You may be scared, but his worst fears have come to pass as well. He may get little or no support from anyone other than you. Here are some more supportive ideas and words you should consider:

a. Empathize: Empathy is the concerted effort to gain an accurate perception of another's experience, and then to share that perception in one's own words. Let them talk, and try to "actively listen" by reflecting back what you hear in your own words.

b. Non-judgmental: Try to focus in on the issue at hand and remove the element of judgment, either positive or negative. It is not your task to determine whether the person being helped is functioning "good" or "bad," but rather try to help them and you gain insight into the person's cross-dressing experience.

c. Assume respect: Unconditionally assume the respect of your husband. The action of cross-dressing should not be the only thing that defines him. People are respected, valued, and cared for simply because they are.

d. Focus on Feelings: Look at the experience that the person shares. Do not try and fix or facilitate "help" for your husband who is sharing the experience. Focus on that person's feelings, which will lead you both eventually to the real reasons behind his cross-dressing. Only the person sharing the experience knows what it is until it is shared and understood by the listener.

10. **Should I talk with my pastor about this? Perhaps he can talk some sense into him?**

A: It is important to seek help, however most ministers will not be thinking of your husband's, yours or your family's welfare. They will be more concerned with the impact it will have on the church. Unfortunately, any help your pastor may want to offer may have his agenda attached to it. There are some very good and understanding ministers out there but most have no experience with transgender issues, and it may not be fair to ask them to make a judgment.

If you want or need to talk with a clergy, you should talk with someone from another congregation who has no ties with your church.

Do not make this a general prayer request. You may not be able to be fix the damage that is done. The best course of action is to contact a neutral trained therapist or seek out a support group.

11. **What is going to happen to the life I thought we both wanted?**

A: This was one of the main reasons why you may not have been previously told about his cross-dressing. He also did not know what would happen to your relationship. He is sharing with you now because he wants the relationship to move forward. It is up to the two of you to determine what the future will bring. I know that this will be a bit scary, but for those who have worked this out together as a couple the rewards are usually worth it.

Andropause – Am I Going Nuts?

While the church was looking the other way, gender issues became much more complex. The simple arguments based on Deuteronomy 22:5 don't begin to touch the reality of what trans individuals deal with. The state of frustration with one's body that a cross-dresser may feel is not natural or Biblically normal.

In Ephesians 5:29, we read:

> *"...no one ever hated his own flesh but nourishes and cherishes it, just as Christ also does the church, because we are members of His body..."*

As we see in scripture, the normal way to think about our bodies is to cherish them. At what point in our lives did we deviate away from this positive and thankful view of our bodies? We need to reverse this downward slide by pursuing real health and this includes an honest look at how our bodies are changing.

"No, but you may be going through Andropause."

In a nutshell, when a man (usually between the ages of 35 and 60) goes through the change of life called andropause, his testosterone level decreases while the estrogen percentage increases. He becomes less aggressive and more gender neutral or softer in his actions and interests. This happens to all males to varying degrees.

Much has been discussed in terms of female menopause, and many books have been written on how to cope with this condition. However, the male counterpart to menopause - andropause - has not been discussed much. Most men have never even heard the term andropause. Although this affects every male to some extent, the medical community is just now beginning to address this condition. Of course, their information is more clinical and scientific, however there is a profound psychological aspect to andropause that still needs to be unpacked.

Most have heard the term mid-life crisis. The man goes out and buys the red sports car or takes up with a woman half his age. Even if there is no outward manifestation, all men deal with growing older and the questions that inevitably follow. Who am I? What have I done with my life? Is this the life that I want? These questions come out of a sense that time is running out, but are heightened by a change in body chemistry. That change in body chemistry is now known as andropause.

Most men are taught to be self-reliant and to "ask for directions" is often viewed as a last resort. However, consider for a moment the teen going through puberty. This would not be a good time to leave a person alone in their thoughts, nor ask them to go through that period of their life without a road map, nor any idea on why they feel the way they do. It would not be the best time for the teen to make life-changing important decisions. A teen going through puberty needs the advice, comfort and protection of family and friends to ease the transition into adulthood.

Unfortunately, an adult male going through andropause is almost always left on their own without any clue as to what is happening to their bodies. They know that something is different, but the support systems are not in place to help them through this significant change of life. Rather than embracing this time as another natural experience and honesty dealing with who they are becoming, men will try to stay it off by using drugs like Viagra, or will seek out testosterone injections. Most men however, are unaware that their bodies are naturally changing and will look outside of themselves for answers to why they feel the way they do.

For those men who have struggled with gender all their lives, during andropause these feelings of confusion can come back with a vengeance. Many men (dealing with gender identity) when they were younger joined the military, pursued the macho job or got married believing that those choices would help them fit into society and that over time the feelings and desires for the feminine would lessen and be more manageable. For some, it is a rude awakening to find out that those feelings actually increase rather than decrease. This often creates frustration and despair. This condition is sometimes referred to as "mid-life crisis."

Usually about the time when andropause starts, the children (if they have any) are grown up and gone, and there is more time to ponder the big questions: Who am I? What have I done with my life? What am I missing? Is this who I want to be? The issue of gender identity at this time often comes back with great force and takes center stage in a person's mind. These individuals are not driven to buy the little red sports car but rather the little red pumps. They may even begin to rewrite their life making a case for extreme change declaring that they never felt okay in their male persona, and that they have no choice but to make a profound change in their gender.

Fueled by hormonal change and a conviction that time is running out, they cross-dress in more earnest. The release and excitement of this sort of feminine exploration may be very intoxicating and feel like a genuine choice or solution to their mid-life struggles. For some, this will lead to pursuing the feminine role full-time through hormones, prolonged periods of cross-dressing and even sexual reassignment surgery (SRS). The latter is sometimes prescribed as a remedy for GID. In offering choices, the medical community does not factor in as much as it should the reality of andropause (mid-life crisis). Often an older man will be asked to make life altering choices in regards to relationships, job, or self-identity when they are biologically in the worst place to do so. Some who make significant changes at this time in their life go on to live very good lives, while others when their hormones level off, see those choices as profoundly wrong in hindsight. It is always best to take it slow through these transitions and not rush into a life-altering change. Seek good professional, psychological and medical support before pursuing any life changing alterations.

As with most choices in life, there are many paths. Some choices are under your control while others are overwhelmingly compelling or completely out of your control.

What is key to good mental health, and to making the best long-term choice possible, is to look at your options and desires in an honest and open manner. Face the reality of what is happening now and be patient for change. Find a trusted person to walk through this time of life with and do not attempt to go through this alone.

Andropause is marked by a decrease in testosterone, so naturally the medical community prescribes increasing artificially the testosterone levels as a treatment. The Harry Benjamin Standard of Care prescribes the female hormone, estrogen, as a treatment for gender identity disorder. Light in the Closet does not advocate either of these treatments as an across-the-board remedy for ALL those dealing with gender identity issues. There are significant health risks associated with both and still a lot of questions around their use. Do not rush into any treatment option without all the facts.

Our bodies change over time and some of that change is natural and should be embraced for what it is. However, there are psychological considerations as well, and for some the potential benefits are worth the physical risks.

Many who have received either testosterone or estrogen treatments report that those treatments have worked well for them - others have had problems.

Why Do I Cross-dress?

Insights and Comments from 12 Cross-dressers

Many men who cross-dress are not even sure why they do. Although the feelings are strong and compelling, the reason or the catalyst as to the "why" is elusive. Most are not able to articulate much beyond some vague compelling feeling. "It just feels good" or "I feel like the real me while cross-dressing" are the most common reasons given to family and friends as to why a person would pursue this expression. However, there is a concrete and knowable reality behind the need for genetic males to express the feminine through cross-dressing, even if they themselves are not aware of it. They range from curiosity and sexual stimulation, to gender identity and even, in rare cases, mental illness. Some explore the opposite gender as a way to connect with suppressed emotions. Others use cross-dressing (CDing) to experience a different life-perspective. The one thing most all cross-dressers have in common is that the need is neither frivolous, nor easily dismissed.

To help understand the mind-set of a cross-dresser, I have solicited the thoughts of twelve people who identify as transgender. None of those surveyed deal with serious mental illness. All those participating would be considered fairly mainstream. All live the bulk of their day as male, or what is referred to as "in male-mode." Most of their friends and family members are unaware of their need to cross-dress. In other words, they would appear to most in society as "normal, upstanding male citizens." All identify as Christian, and most are either leaders or active members in their perspective churches.

Those who provided comments share a few things in common:

1. They all questioned the act of CDing as to its morality in light of cultural and scriptural concerns.

2. They all tried in earnest to fight or shutdown their feelings and stop CDing at one time or another.

3. They have all struggled with this since a young age (before the age of 8 years) and have never been able to free themselves from their CDing needs, desires or thoughts.

4. They all sought some form of professional counseling, or reparative therapy. This resulted in an increased understanding of the subject, but not a relief from its hold.

5. They all experienced, through acceptance of their transgender condition, a certain amount of peace and relief from guilt. Their feminine expression ranges from a total embrace of CDing, to a limited occasional activity.

6. Even after decades, the feelings for most are stronger now than in their youth, and the issue of desiring to express the feminine is very active. Some identify fully as female, while others would place themselves along some point on the gender spectrum. They range in age from 40-85 years.

Below are quotes from these twelve cross-dressers. They offer a range of thoughts and experiences. These comments are unedited.

Quotes from MS - "Mary"

"When cross-dressed, I became wrought with shame in my teenage years, but now working through this struggle, it has become a badge of courage. As a productive senior citizen, I tend now to follow my heart and am not afraid, like I used to be, to enter areas that are labeled "Do Not Enter" by my local community. Dealing with this condition has given me courage."

"Who do I hurt by cross-dressing? I definitely hurt the feelings of those of my family who fear the repercussions from some in my local community if they ever found out. It seems to me that I mostly offend the person who fears that they may be transgender or even gay themselves."

"By my cross-dressing I seek not to endanger any person. I seek only to discover more of myself and to create a safe environment to experiment in."

Quotes from JM - "Natalie"

"When I dress as a woman I am expressing the maternal softness and vulnerability that I find within myself (softness that I usually conceal and am embarrassed of). I cross-dressed, instinctively in my youth and then purposely in my senior years, to form a more perfect union of all that is me."

"I know the peace of God and I know it well and I have been privileged to experience his supernatural calmness and encouragement often. The thing is, I have never experienced His peace when I have been cross-dressed or even when contemplating doing it."

Quotes from RS - "Jennifer"

"I do not believe God leads me to cross-dress or that He made me transgender. In other words, the reason He never speaks to me about CDing may be that He isn't leading me to do it. Having said that, however, I must quickly confess that a part of me greatly enjoys cross-dressing and exploring life as a woman. God does not condone or condemn my CDing in its entirety. There are many aspects to my CDing. These can be both good and bad — both hurtful and healthy. God did not preordain my transgender nature, but He did allow for it, and so is able to redeem it. God did not ordain my gender confusion or the rigid social gender roles I have to contend with. He has used my CDing though, as an opportunity to teach me."

"Perhaps I do not have the peace I seek for, because God does not intend for me to stop my exploration yet. He has more for me to learn. Perhaps cross-dressing is not intended to give me peace, but instead to spur me on towards discovery, and hopefully a healthy self-image?"

"Maybe CDing has caused me to throw myself at the Lord more than I otherwise would have."

Quotes from BM - "Still deciding on female persona"

"It's a complicated issue and the most troubling of any in my life. I have told the Lord many times that it won't change unless He does something about it, for apparently I am unwilling or unable to do much about it on my own. Why is that? I don't know but that is the question I'm dealing with and prayerfully I will get somewhere with it. I now rely on God to change my heart and desires as He sees fit. Not in a passive way, but in a guilt-free expectant way."

"I want to ask myself, 'Is being a cross-dresser and all of the thoughts, feelings and attitudes I have, made me more like the person I would like to be or less?' The answer is a resounding "no." No, I do not like being a person with what is, to some extent, a secret life and to be so absorbed in that. I do not like the constant secrecy, lying and battling that goes on with all of this -- it is not good to live a lie or a double life. However, I suppose I play many different roles daily as I find the need. Obviously, my cross-dressing is a big role change, more so than most. However, I also have my church face, my game face, my husband face, my son face, my dad face, and my private face. These may look somewhat the same, but there are still differences. Each face I wear has an exposed side and another I choose to hide. Perhaps this is a lie, perhaps not. I think I can get frustrated and falter if my secrecy leads to guilt. When I hide too much of who I am, my relationships are jeopardized."

"Why would anyone choose to go against society, religion, biology, and psychology to live even momentarily as something they're obviously not, if there was not a compelling reason to do so? It requires such an enormous suspension of reality for me to do this. Only a strong motivation like sexual pleasure could cause my behavior. So, is this just sexual? I went to sex addicts anonymous, and tried to work through their "12" steps. I realized that this was not it. I liked sex as much as anyone else, maybe more than some, but I don't need to dress like a woman to find sexual pleasure."

"Five years of counseling and reparative therapy turned up nothing.

I tried, yes, I even hoped and prayed I could find something to point to and thus find healing from cross-dressing. I tried to blame mom and dad for some repressed childhood trauma, but found nothing there either. Mom and Dad weren't perfect, but they were about as normal for post-WWII parents as you could imagine. I've since met with many other men who struggled with various adult addictions and these guys had some really bad parenting, yet not one was interested in cross-dressing. The childhood abuse or trauma argument just did not apply to me."

Quotes from DJ - "Kathy"

"I cross-dressed and then went back to "normal." I envied women (their beauty and appeal) but I didn't idolize them. Becoming a complete-woman was not my goal. CDing is only an occasional crutch to deal with pain and stress."

"Considering my people pleasing personality, my need to CD must be something very strong to make me risk the wrath and ridicule of family, friends, and society in general. It was more than curiosity and relaxation. I welcomed the relief at finally being real and honest. CDing is not a desperate attempt to escape reality. It feels right and comfortable. I feel real."

Quotes from NP - "Diane"

"Was I a closeted homosexual? I gave it my best shot, but just could not find any desire for men of any type. In fact, physical closeness to men repulses me."

"It's as if my brain is somehow hard-wired to be a woman in spite of my chromosomes and genitalia, in spite of being raised as a boy, in spite of being successful as a man, husband, father, and grandfather. Whatever makes someone feel like a man or woman must exist in the brain and not just the organs and hormones. This was the only way I could explain my desires and thoughts."

Quotes from ER - "Silome"

"My exploration of being transgender has led me to conclude that I was fearfully and wondrously made by God; He knit me together in my mother's womb; He made me the way I am for His glory and to enjoy Him forever. Years of constant daily prayer for the truth have given me no other answer. Realizing I am who I am, transgender, has given me much comfort."

"It was only after I became aware of other trans persons, that I stopped to examine my life and began to recognize a pattern of behavior that indicated an unusual comfort with the feminine role. As I embraced this just a little, it opened up a flood of emotions I never expected or sought. It was like being honest and real for the first time in my life. So why not embrace this and transition to living as a woman? The cost of that is high by all accounts, very high. I'm not willing to pay that price. I don't want to give up my family and friends and I feel I would have to. I'm not even sure I would want to live full time as a woman if I could. I'm also comfortable living as a man; whether this is due to long practice or the wiring of my brain, I'm not sure. I suspect the latter, though. I envision gender as a continuum and I'm somewhere very near the mid point of it."

Quotes from Margie

"Whenever possible, I present as a woman as completely as a 6 foot 2 inch frame allows. I don't sense I'm acting or putting on so much as I'm allowing myself to be and express what has been long suppressed. Life is not perfect, but it is good."

"I do not consider 'it' cross-dressing. I don't feel women's clothing is not the opposite gender for me, but my normal way of dressing."

"I certainly have emotional needs, but I am an engineer with a master's degree and am a scientist at heart, so I need to understand the clinical side of this as well. This should go a long way to dispelling much of the "out of hand" dismissal of my ultraconservative church background. I am only recently out to my wife of 40 years and she is struggling with this mightily. I don't see myself as ever transitioning but being TG is an undeniable part of me that needs to be recognized and accommodated. My two selves are very separate and I have no immediate plans to share this information with my current church. They would not necessarily be judgmental, it's just that I don't want to go through all of that if I don't have to."

Quotes from MM - "Sheri"

"This morning, in a very clear way, while I was cross-dressing the Lord imparted to me the gift of no condemnation. For the first time ever, I have the peace of God while cross-dressed. This is a very big deal."

"I worry about people finding out. I don't know what they would think. If I were to ask any number of people in my office, for example, what they think of Christians I suspect I'd hear adjectives used like narrow-minded, hypocritical, homophobic, misogynistic and intolerant. In my experience at least, those adjectives don't really fit the Christians I know. It isn't who I am as a Christian. I don't think I would fit their image of what a cross-dresser is either."

Quotes from MR - "Janet"

"In high school I was class president, dated the homecoming queen and played football. I'm a college graduate, and I've always had good jobs. I've made a lot of money and have a great family. I've been in many small men's groups at church and have facilitated many too and I have to say I have far less insecurities than most men I know. So it actually still freaks me out to some degree that I want to shave myself and become Janet."

"Maybe I want to cross-dress because it feels safe. When I'm dressed in female attire I feel completely honest. I like how I feel when I'm female... but honestly, I don't dislike how I feel as a guy. I've never suffered from a feeling of loathing of being a man...although I've never been comfortable with some stereotypical guy stuff either. Cross-dressing represents a REAL vacation to me. An opportunity to shed the burdens inherent in my life and temporarily become a softer, more overtly loving version of myself. I often have marveled at how much closer I tend to feel to God while CDing."

"How did I get this way? My parents, God love them, were so hilariously hyper vigilant about gender roles and behavior that almost anything but anger and exaltation were labeled "feminine." If I cried it was "girlish." If I expressed tenderness demonstratively or wanted to learn to cook I was acting girly, and that was a bad thing. Cross-dressing became the method I used to reclaim that which God wanted to originally give me."

Quotes from JC - "Lori"

"I'm finally learning to accept that this is my "thorn in the flesh"...and that that's okay. I actually find myself looking forward to my future!"

"Having spent 45 years in the evangelical church, I have always been under the bondage that what I am doing will send me to hell. Now, in recent months I have stopped fighting who I am. I have even begun praying as Lori, and was shocked to feel totally at peace with that. It is hard to accept that after a lifetime of my femininity being sin to me that I can still communicate with God while expressing my feminine side. I'm afraid though that if my family learns of this they will think that I am headed for hell. I know what people say about being surprised at who accepts you, and a Gender Therapist I consulted suggested that two of my children might understand. However, I am not sure since I see how negative they are towards the homosexuals in our family. I really want to socialize as Lori. I keep telling myself that if Lori must go away for my family's sake, that I want to at least have socialized as Lori a few times. I plan to find a support group."

Quotes from SP - "Carol"

"I asked myself why I wanted to go out as a woman. Searching my heart for an answer, I found it was simply what I wanted to do. My guy side can't understand this need, but the fem part laughs and says, 'What else did you expect?' So here I am, so unsure, searching for truth from God and myself, while all along walking on a road that I walk involuntarily."

"This road has been difficult, but the growth, life lessons, self-acceptance, peace, grace, and physical health I have received through acceptance is very much a redemptive act. God did not "heal" me of what I thought was an affliction, but instead used it in a redemptive way. He redeemed who I am, rather than change me into someone else."

"It is hard to attach blame on someone else for my CDing. I don't think it was any one thing that makes me want to cross-dress. All I know is that when I stopped struggling and began to accept myself, the desire to dress became manageable. Accepting my needs, freed me from guilt"

"My wife has been very understanding of my need to express the feminine side of me, and both of us know when I need a break from my "male" life. This is all still new to me, but I think I am beginning to understand why I feel the way I do. I'm glad I have someone to share this gender identity issue with who is not judgmental."

Why We Cross-dress - A list of Reasons and Catalysts

1. **Child abuse (emotional and physical)**

   Both physical and emotional abuse, especially from a trusted adult, are destructive actions that victimizes the child. Abuse leaves lasting marks which if not addressed, can affect the quality of life for the survivor well into adulthood. The act of abuse often leaves the victim feeling out-of-control. Cross-dressing can be a way to cope with the emotional pain of past child abuse. It can be a way to attempt to regain control. The endorphins released during cross-dressing and the comfort of the clothing can help to relax and center and can be used as a type of therapy, or self-medication in some cases. Someone who is abused may turn to cross-dressing for comfort, but cross-dressing is rarely the direct result or response to abuse. Rather, a more purely fetish behavior will often be embraced by the victim of abuse. Usually a specific object or objects are fixated on that represent the actions of the abuser. This fetish component could be incorporated into a person's cross-dressing, but only a trained therapist with knowledge of both abuse and gender identity can sort this out.

2. **Gender-related Taunting**

   Although not as prevalent with today's youth, many boys have been victims of gender taunting. Some boys identify more with girls and feel more comfortable around their female peers. When a boy demonstrates female tendencies, expressions or interests, he might become a victim of taunting. If ostracized by his male peers, this disassociation with the male gender could become a catalyst for a boy to experiment with cross-dressing. He may develop a close association and connection with his female image. The person who is the object of persistent gender-related taunting almost always has demonstrated those feminine characteristics being cited by his peers. Taunting may drive a boy to choose the female over the male, but the desire to be female usually already exists.

   Not all boys turn-away from their taunting male peers. A boy, who wishes to fit in, may succumb to the taunting and deny himself those feminine interests cited by his peers, or try and cease his feminine expressions or change his mannerisms. This will almost always result in emotional damage, and a poor self-image.

3. **Emotional Gender Identity**

   There is a distinctive difference between the typical male and female brains. Some biological males are born with what is considered a more typically "female brain" as evidenced by emotional responses and self-declared interests. Many cross-dressers consider this condition as their most important reason to express themselves in the female mode. Powerful emotions while cross-dressed come to the surface of even the most placid male. These feelings can preoccupy much of the cross-dresser's day, even when they are in male mode. The reason for this may be biological or sociological. Both are valid, real, and need to be recognized.

4. **Biologically Pseudo-female or Androgynous Body Type**

   There is a wide gender spectrum of body types, emotions and interests. Many who cross-dress are expressing not only how they feel mentally, but are responding to what their body is telling them physically. Some males have body types that could be confused for female. Wide hips, enlarged chests or breast, and small hands to name a few. Some males simply do not feel comfortable in male clothing; it really does not fit them well. They may have a healthy self-image and truly feel more comfortable expressing themselves as female or softer in appearance. Often these males will adopt a more androgynous look. Some may even consider themselves as "inter-sexed" even though the sexual organs may not be ambiguous.

5. **Psychological Female Gender Identity**

   This is often the most common reason for a male to dress as a female. Regardless of the catalyst, someone who has chosen cross-dressing to express an inner need will usually have a psychological profile showing that they have a strong alignment to female sensitivities or typically female thought patterns. Most males in our society have very rigid ideas about what is and is not allowed for a male to express. These males while cross-dressed, give themselves permission to embrace their inherent female psychological make up and express the feelings they deny themselves in male mode. Our sociological conditioning is such that many males find it impossible to express these emotions and thoughts unless they are cross-dressed.

6. **Social Gender Identity**

   A male may cross-dress as a woman to join in social activities that interest "her" which "he" has previously suppressed or avoided because of social gender roles. The desire to experience social situations as female will often lead a cross-dresser to join social groups. Activities and social settings include dining out, shopping, playing sports, or just taking long walks. Sometimes a cross-dresser will want to partake in other typically female roles while "dressed" including, cleaning the home, cooking and gardening.

7. **Fetish**

   Some use cross-dressing as a tool to express fetish behavior. This however usually includes some sort of object for sexual stimulation that is not inherently related to sexual function. Most fetish behavior focuses on a specific aspect of clothing such as shoes. Also role playing, wearing seductive costumes, or dressing in tightly constricting clothing can be a fetish expression of sorts. But not all these have a clinical or psychological root in fetish behavior, and the person may just be cross-dressing for fun or curiosity. A true fetish behavior is often a result of childhood trauma.

8. **Depression**

Although not a reason to cross-dress, it can be a catalyst. The act of cross-dressing can release endorphins that are shown to help battle depression. Although these endorphins can sometimes become addictive, much like someone who is a runner or jogger becomes addicted to the runners high, cross-dressing can be an effective tool for self-medication.

9. **Chronic Depression**

Much like regular momentary depression, the endorphin rush experienced through cross-dressing can ease the symptoms of chronic depression. However, the effects are very short term and not as profound. Chronic depression is much more severe, and only an aggressive treatment program including therapy and chemical aids can offer real effective chronic depression management.

10. **Fun/Entertainment**

For some cross-dressing is just a costume and used as play. These males still relate strongly to their male role but just wish to express an aspect of the feminine, or mimic women for a short time.

11. **Curiosity or Envy**

People are normally very curious. Some males want to see what it would be like to be in the role of a woman. If this is the main reason to cross-dress the act of cross-dressing is short-lived. Envy is included in this category because both do not have a long-term, biological, sociological or psychological component. A cross-dresser may say that they envy or idolize a woman's body, but this, by itself is not a compelling reason to cross-dress.

12. **Relieve Stress**

Some feel extreme pressure in their everyday or "male" lives. The act of wearing women's clothes allows a male to take a break from their social masculine expectations, restrictions or pressures. Cross-dressing for these males is escapism.

13. **Poor Male Self-Image/Acceptance**

Some males wish to escape their male image because of a negative or poor self-image. Although most were well adjusted when toddlers or even young boys, they become increasingly disassociated or disconnected from their male persona and male peers as they age. Those boys who are not gender-polarized towards the male end of the spectrum may find it hard to fit in with other boys. This lack of acceptance can lead to the development of a poor self-image. They often feel as if they have no real male friends and will gravitate toward a female expression in hopes for some peer acceptance. An affirming transgender community is often the only community they may feel comfortable with. Although not a reason to begin cross-dressing, it is a compelling one to continue. Affirmation of their feminine image by others can help improve a negative self-image.

14. Andropause / Mid-life Crisis

When a man (usually between the ages of 35 and 60) goes through the change of life, it is called andropause. At this time, testosterone levels decrease while the estrogen percentage increases. He becomes less aggressive and more gender neutral or softer in his actions and interests. This happens to all males to varying degrees. If he has previously demonstrated a desire or a proclivity to cross-dress, the hormonal changes during andropause can be a catalyst to begin cross-dressing again in earnest. This is sometimes referred to as mid-life crisis. Who am I? What have I done with my life? Is this the life that I want? These questions come out of a sense that time is running out, but are heightened by a change in the body's chemistry. A drop in testosterone may make a male feel more feminine, and re-ignite a desire to look and act more female.

15. Sexual Expression

We are sexual beings, and the act of cross-dressing can release powerful sexual emotions, making it easier for some men to connect with their feelings. Sexual orientation usually is unaffected.

16. Schizophrenia / Mental Illness

Decades ago, the diagnosis for being transsexual or transgender was mental disorder. Schizophrenia was the most common diagnosis, since the person who was male was declaring himself to be female. This was mistakenly interpreted as having two personalities. This condition was considered a serious illness needing therapy, including shock therapy. However, this was almost always a misdiagnosis in that a transgender person is aware of their choice, and has purposed to pursue it in order to develop congruent personhood.

Fortunately, the medical community today sees the "schizophrenia" diagnosis as unsubstantiated in all but some very rare cases. However, with many cross-dressers, the alternative "female" personality is a distinctly different persona from their male. "She" frequently has "her" own name and social niche. Rather than being a mental disorder, this double-life is often a matter of convenience for associating with other cross-dressers. For some this alternative personality could even have "a life of her own." This is not, however, a split personality because the cross-dresser knows that the "female" character is in addition to their male persona, and is aware of the distinction. An individual with true schizophrenia or a mental disorder has a break with the reality of their situation and could have more than two personas.

This individual should seek clinical help for their condition.

17. **Inter-sexed or Hermaphrodite**

Some people are born inter-sexed and their choice of clothing or gender expression can confuse others as to how they wish to be related to since their gender is non-specific.

Their choice of clothing should never be considered cross-dressing, but just a declaration of personhood. Often their clothing choice is gender non-specific as well.

18. **Personal Choice/Drag**

Some call their cross-dressing a hobby that occupies their leisure time. They have no real underlying psychological reason to cross-dress. They dress in women's clothes purely as a creative or fun outlet. "I just feel like it" is reason enough for them. A male who dresses in drag to entertain does not usually identify as a cross-dresser or transgender in terms of their gender identity, but refer to themselves as female impersonators, or drag queens.

19. **Cross-gender Predisposition**

All those who identify as transgender and use cross-dressing to connect with a gender have a predisposition to do so. Whether it is nurture, nature or choice, or a combination of all three, the desire to be living as female is a predisposition. This is not a fully conscious or personal choice on their part, but goes deep into the core of how they relate to the world. The feminine form feels real and authentic because it is.

This list is not all-inclusive but touches on many of the reasons why a male may want to look like and be treated as female. Those who cross-dress when younger as experimentation may continue as the get older or may cease. Sometimes a person who is trans may stop their cross-dressing experimentation during their teenage years. The natural female tendencies, however, will remain even if those feelings are being denied. Severe anger, depression or even thoughts of self-injury may result if suppressing female desires and emotions is due to outside oppression.

It is important to look at the mental, emotional and physical health over the idea of right and wrong when supporting a trans youth. Cross-dressing can be good therapy for physical and psychological alignment.

Education and Research

There has been a lot of education and new research regarding transgender issues in recent years. Research into causes and treatments are being perused by clinicians, medical institutions, universities, and schools. In 2010 in the United States, the concept of someone identifying as transgender was still new, and its introduction into society moved forward with little debate. The trans community was able to work with doctors, religious leaders, and politicians to help develop inclusion in faith communities, education in schools, and accessible healthcare. National events to support the transgender community were multiplying throughout the US. Those who may have opposed the trans community ignored it for the most part since it was so small, and was not on the radar of most people.

Then in 2015 there was push back both politically and socially. Inroads into the medical and educational system were being view as a breakdown of American family values. When President Trump took office in 2016 he made it his mission to disenfranchise the trans community and oppose it at every turn. He encouraged legislation to limit transgender healthcare, participation in sports, access to social services, housing, employment, civil rights, and more. In his second term in 2024, he sought to expunge the word transgender and delete our very existence. He required his followers to rally against the trans community. Over 2,000 state and federal anti-trans bills were introduced between the years 2024 to 2026. Hundreds of those have passed, and in some states the trans community has been criminalized.

Even so, there are loud voices that continue to fight for the rights and even the very existence of those children of God who identify as transgender.

Light in the Closet has been part of that fight since 2008 and will continue to speak up and not be silenced.

Living an Integrated Life

God desires us to be honest. God has paved for us an accessible path so that we might follow Christ with our whole heart, mind and spirit.

For us to be effective in Christian service we should be fully integrated people. All aspects of our personality should be open and subject to the authority of God. When we hide a secret, or live a double life, we close off the power of God to move within us, which greatly cripples our ability to follow God. Confessing our sins, shortcomings, and struggles to God and to each other is important if we are to pursue a grace-filled, abundant life. In the book, *Speaking the Truth in Love - How to be an Assertive Christian*, by Ruth Koch and Kenneth Haugk, the authors state:

> "Of course the fully integrated personality is the ideal. Human beings are all less than fully integrated. In fact, one of the life tasks for everyone is to move in the direction of more fully integrating all the separate components of his or her personality... What was whole at creation was broken and fragmented by sin, and Jesus has come personally into history and into individual lives to restore wholeness...God is willing to supply, through the power of the Holy Spirit, the wholeness that you need."

Confessing struggles, weaknesses and failings, and pursuing self-acceptance is critical to becoming a fully integrated person.

Baby and Bath Water

You've heard it said, "Don't throw the baby out with the bath water!" We were created as we are for the purpose of glorifying God. Just because we desire to change, it does not automatically follow that change should occur, or is even healthy for us. Those personality traits or quirks that we consider to be weaknesses are a necessary part of what we would consider our personality strengths. It is difficult to stuff into our emotional closets one specific "undesirable" aspect of our personalities. Unfortunately, those who try to do so often end up shutting down completely. We may be able to, for a time, squelch certain undesirable actions or expressions. However frustration will usually result because we have no healthy outlet to express that part of our authentic selves. Real psychological needs must have some form of release for us to be psychologically and physically healthy.

Without the comfort and encouragement of others, we can end up trapped in a bitter cycle of indulgence, stifling guilt, repentance, frustration and back to indulgence. We continue in this cycle because the underlying personality issues and needs are never addressed. No matter what we try, our true basic personality remains unaltered.

If we view our weaknesses only stumbling blocks to spiritual growth, we won't honestly deal with those weaknesses but instead we'll stuff them into the back of our closets. Ignoring an issue denies us the opportunity to deal with that issue honestly. However, our weaknesses if confronted, can lead to realistic self-evaluation, Godly understanding, and positive growth. Our weaknesses can draw us closer to others in our faith communities for mutual support. This process will help us draw closer to God and the divine within us.

Sometimes our weaknesses and struggles are there for a reason. As Paul wrote to the Corinthian church:

> *"To keep me from becoming conceited...there was given me a thorn in my flesh...Three times I pleaded with the Lord to take it away from me. But He said to me, "My grace is sufficient for you, for my power is made perfect in weakness." Therefore I will boast all the more gladly about my weaknesses, so that Christ's power may rest on me. (2 Corinthians 12:7-9)*

We need to rely on the grace God provides. This grace allows us to express ourselves and discover who we are without the threat of a broken relationship with our Creator. The pursuit of an integrated life allows us to develop real relationships that include our whole being.

Jesus went to the cross, not to appease God, but to demonstrate how far God will go to connect with us in a way we will understand.

Avoiding Cultural Judgments and Pursuing God's Righteousness

The righteousness of man should never be confused with the righteousness of God. Unfortunately our understanding of God and scripture is filtered through our personal experiences. As a result, we usually make judgments of others based on our cultural comfort zone. As Christians, we have the duty and honor to speak and act on behalf of God. So, when we have the opportunity to show Christ to others, we should avoid applying our own righteous standards to that person. Our judgment of others, in effect, minimizes the righteousness of God, lowering God to our level. It is not our place to judge another person's standing before God, but with humility we are called to serve one another in faith and love.

Romans 10: 1, 3-13 discusses pitfalls concerning culturally-driven standards of righteousness, and the temptation to pass judgment on another's eternal standing:

> *"...For not knowing about God's righteousness and seeking to establish their own, they did not subject themselves to the righteousness of God. For Christ is the end of the law of righteousness to everyone who believes. For Moses writes that the man who practices the righteousness which is based on law shall live by that righteousness."* (This man is living by his own standard and not God's standard.)
>
> *"But the righteousness based on faith speaks as follows: "DO NOT SAY IN YOUR HEART, 'WHO WILL ASCEND INTO HEAVEN?'* (that is, to bring Christ down)*, or 'WHO WILL DESCEND INTO THE ABYSS?'."* (that is, to bring Christ up from the dead) But what does it say? *"THE WORD IS NEAR YOU, IN YOUR MOUTH AND IN YOUR HEART"* – that is, the word of faith which we are preaching, that if you confess with your mouth Jesus as Lord, and believe in your heart that God raised Him from the dead, you will be saved; for with the heart a person believes, resulting in righteousness, and with the mouth he confesses, resulting in salvation.
>
> For the Scripture says, *"WHOEVER BELIEVES IN HIM WILL NOT BE DISAPPOINTED." "For there is no distinction between Jew and Greek; for the same Lord is Lord of all, abounding in riches for all who call on Him..."*

The world too often bears witness to the hypocrisy of a church that defines certain actions as sins, yet practices and excuses their own shortcomings. Some "sins" are allowed within the Church walls and freely discussed, while other "sins" are never mentioned. It is apparent that the church often operates under a hierarchy of sin.

The sins or actions we are able to understand, and tolerate in others, are those we share in common with them. If we share in a struggle then we are more sympathetic to that struggle. If we do not share in someone's struggle we will have no understanding of what they are going through and little tolerance for that person. The church should be the one place where diversity should be expressed and we are accepted as we are.

Christ set us free from the power of sin. This statement is often mistaken as a call to "clean-up" our act. The power that sin has over us is not in the doing of the sin. The real power of sin comes from shifting our focus off of grace and onto a legalistic obsession over *what is or isn't sin*. If we obsess over legalism then "sin" has set our agenda, not grace. Fear of negative consequences can preoccupy our thoughts and drive our agendas. If our lives are controlled by a list of "don'ts" (don't do this, or that), then we are not enjoying the freedom from sin that Christ offers. Freedom from sin inspires us to pursue those callings God has put on our hearts. A renewed life is not one controlled by a laundry list of don'ts. Prayer and the pursuit of God become the focus when we stop obsessing over self-justification.

1 Corinthians 15:56-57 helps us understand that the power sin has over us is only understood through the law.

> *"The sting of death is sin, and the power of sin is the law. But thanks be to God! He gives us the victory through our Lord Jesus Christ."*

Our victory in Christ allows us to make realistic self-assessments, and embrace our freedom found in forgiveness. Romans 3:20 makes this bold statement:

> *Therefore no one will be declared righteous in God's sight by the works of the law; rather, through the law we become conscious of our sin."*

Our freedom in Christ comes when we admit our shortcomings without condemning ourselves. The law is a tool to *refine* us rather than *define* us. Take your focus off what your consider to be sin, and instead practice the grace-filled fruits of the spirit: peace, patience, kindness, joy, goodness, faithfulness, gentleness, self-control, and, most importantly, love. This leads to a peace and purpose that will resonate in your divine nature.

Missing Grace in the Conservative Church

"I did not leave the Church, the Church left me."

Growing up in the conservative church I heard the message of grace preached from the pulpit and reiterated in the Sunday school classroom. The teachings of Jesus and the way he lived his life was held up as a standard to aspire to. Love, self-sacrifice, honesty, truthfulness, patience, kindness, gentleness, and empathy were promoted as good traits and a way-of-life to be embrace. Identifying fundamental Christian virtues in the lifestyle and actions of a leader, (love, joy, peace, patience, kindness, goodness, faithfulness, gentleness, and self-control) was vital when choosing those whom we should follow.

I grew up believing, that the pursuit of spiritual fruit needed to frame the agenda of those in leadership.

Yes, my pastors and teachers were not perfect, but it was assumed that they strive to include these attributes and actions in their lives. It is what I looked for in my parents and those whose authority I was under. Knowing my leaders were attempting to live this way gave me confidence that I was on the right path as I engaged in Christian community.

I still believe that this sort of life direction is God's will for all God's children.

The Biblical book of Matthew states that "we" will know "them" (those who claim faith) by their fruit.[1] It reads that a good tree will produce good fruit and that a bad tree will produce bad fruit. If someone exhibits the fruit of the Spirit (love, joy, peace, patience, kindness, goodness, faithfulness, gentleness, and self-control)[2] they have demonstrated that they are followers of the Christian doctrine and of Christ. If these attributes and actions were not exhibited, then that person was unworthy of the Christian leadership mantle. I embraced this as an obvious truth. Pursuing the fruits of the spirit in my own life is what brought me to my knees and what also raised me up in hope. I assumed that I was part of a community who all sought after the same thing. Jesus was my standard and my guide, and although I came up short, I trusted that those who I shared a pew with felt and believed as I did.

To identify and encourage the ripening of the "fruits of the spirit" in others is a unifying mandate from God for the Church. This agenda of grace and hope is illuminated through demonstrations of inclusion and kindness. Honesty and integrity are critically important for any real growth of the spirit. Being fearless in the pursuit of Christ, even when it is uncomfortable or risky, is necessary for any real spiritual growth.

I still believe this to be true, even though the church I grew up in, and trusted to promote these ideals and attributes, apparently does not value them as it once did.

What the many conservative churches promote today (through fear and mistrust of others) is an agenda of exclusion and judgment. The focus has shifted off the fruits of the spirit and onto a mission of weeding out unrighteousness. These churches use a patched together pseudo-Christian morality to identify those they wish to vilify and ostracize. Preaching division from the pulpit by identifying "who the enemy is" has underlined their agendas and teachings. Real Christian love and acceptance is not embraced as a necessary part of the church's message. They refuse to include even those with a strong moral code who identify as Christian, if they are also gay, lesbian, transgender, or queer (among others). These Christians are viewed by them as unacceptable for inclusion in their community. The conservative church believes it has a duty to judge and condemn those Jesus had, in fact, asked his Church to serve. The church was never intended to be a seat of judgment of others. Jesus asks our focus to be inward, "Why do you look at the speck in your brother's eye, but do not consider the plank in your own eye?"[3]

Why has this shift away from love and grace occurred? I believe that the conservative church is following corrupt and ungodly leaders who exhibit almost none of the fruits of the spirit. It holds up these corrupt leaders as men of God. It declares them to have a mandate from God to weed out undesirables and to build walls and hedges around the physical and emotional comforts they have appropriated for themselves.

The mandates from Jesus are ignored:

Jesus encourages us to be selfless, yet they are self-centered.[4]

Jesus demonstrates compassion for those outside the city walls, yet they lock the doors.[5]

Jesus declares men, women and others to be valid and of equal value, yet they devalue and oppress women and vilify those outside the polarized gender norms.[6]

Jesus teaches that those we follow should be someone who serves others, yet we elect leaders who are self-serving.[7]

Jesus asks for us to encourage temperance and to promote kindness, yet they honor bullies without patience or self-control.[8]

Jesus healed the sick and gave hope to the despondent, yet they turn their back on those who are inconvenient and unprotected.[9]

Jesus reached out to the widows and women who struggled, yet they deny a women's self-determination and devalue her contributions.[10]

Jesus helped the homeless and hungry asking us to give freely, yet they give only scraps while hoarding their possessions in clenched fists. "If there is among you a poor man of your brethren…you shall not harden your heart nor shut your hand from your poor brother, but you shall open your hand wide to him and willingly lend him sufficient for his need, whatever he needs." [11]

Jesus gave as a clear agenda for what God sees as righteousness, yet they have strayed from that path declaring themselves already righteous.

These members in the conservative Christian church are the new Pharisees. What they are doing is not new. There are many throughout spiritual history that have become oppressors. Their agenda of weeding out what they see as evil is not dissimilar to that of today's ultra-conservative Islamic fundamentalists.

They misuse the name of Jesus to promote fear and distrust of those who differ in the slightest from their idols of self-righteousness. They use the threat of hell for those who do not toe the line, declaring certain actions and desires to be outside of grace in order to keep congregants following their agenda.[12]

The runaway train of the conservative Church has derailed the spiritual growth of their members. It's a spiritual train wreck. The Church has unwittingly made itself an adversary of God. Jesus declares, "Woe to you, religious-leaders, hypocrites! For you are like whitewashed tombs which indeed appear beautiful outwardly, but inside are full of dead men's bones and all uncleanness. Woe to you, church-leaders, hypocrites! For you shut up the kingdom of heaven, you neither go in yourselves, nor do you allow those who are supposed to enter to go in."

With all these warnings and clear messages, how is it that the conservative church misses what is fundamentally important? How is it that they hold in high regard those who demonstrate none of the fruits of the spirit? Distrust has replaced inclusion. Hate has been repackaged as integrity and love. Those who bully, and puff themselves up are given places of honor and are celebrated.[13]

When Jesus walked the streets of Jerusalem, he was oppressed by many of the leaders in his day who have now passed their mantle to the conservative Church. Those Pharisees saw Jesus as the enemy because of his radical teachings of inclusion, value, love, self-sacrifice, and his questioning of religious leadership and their misdirected idea of righteousness. Those religious leaders rejected the teachings of Jesus and helped to facilitate his crucifixion.

Today's conservative religious leaders have defined for themselves what a righteous lifestyle looks like and so have oppressed and rejected anyone who does not follow their specific "righteous" model.[14] This oppression is often directed at the single parent, those who are childless, the divorced person (even those escaping abuse), women (especially those who God has called to leadership), the entire LGBTQI++ community (currently focused on the exclusion and oppression of trans people) and anyone else who does not "look" like them.[15] They pick and choose who they will tolerate for inclusion offering a roadmap to congregants that they themselves don't truly follow.[16] Their Bibles have been edited with underlining, while they compile their list of "right and wrong." They chose from a smorgasbord of scriptures, only those verses they can easily stomach.[17]

They have shunned the real meaning of grace which is what all of Jesus's teachings point to; "Grace is the basis for the Christian faith. Grace cannot be earned; it is something that is freely given, it is undeserved favor. Grace is the bridge built for ALL our relationships with God."

The primary focus is no longer on spiritual fruit and encouraging real spiritual growth and awakenings. Instead, the conservative church has become a cultural, social, and political entity that promotes a philosophy and ideology seeking to preserve their institution, customs, values and the status-quo. Jesus spoke out against this 2,000 years ago. Jesus showed us how to speak the truth, even when it brings about conflict. His followers today need to have the courage to do the same.

DON'T GIVE UP – There is Hope

Even though the conservative church has lost its way, there are still Christians, and Christian organizations that are pursuing the fruits of the spirit and echo the heart of God. Some of these are:

Richard Rohr: Richard is a Franciscan friar, and founder of the Center for Action and Contemplation: Father Richard Rohr bears witness to the deep wisdom of Christian mysticism and traditions of action and contemplation.

WEBSITE: cac.org/about/cac-faculty/cac-founder-richard-rohr

Evangelicals for Democracy: "America Needs Help: Evangelicals for Democracy is the first non-partisan, faith-based nonprofit 501(c)3 organization working to empower evangelicals to preserve democracy by seeking the truth and supporting the democratic tenets of our society. Our goal is to build understanding that protecting democracy protects us and our fundamental rights."

WEBSITE: evangelicalsfordemocracy.org

CLGS: Center for LGBTQI+ & Gender Studies in Religion: "The Center for LGBTQI+ and Gender Studies in Religion (CLGS) was established at Pacific School of Religion in Berkeley, California and opened its doors in the fall of 2000. The Center serves three distinct but overlapping constituencies: the world of academic religious scholarship; faith communities; and lesbian, gay, bisexual, queer and transgender people and organizations. For each of these constituent groups, CLGS is committed to providing programming and support for research, resources, education for leadership, and community-building/advocacy."

WEBSITE: clgs.org

Queer Theology: "Queer Theology has developed tons of resources over the years. The resources are organized by topic so you can find exactly what you're looking. Topics like: "Is it's okay to be LGBTQI+" and "Navigating sex and relationships" as well as "Reclaiming the Bible."

WEBSITE: queertheology.com/transgender-christian

These are just some of the hundreds of resources available. I believe we will see many more statements of "true faith" coming to light over the next few months and years as those who wish to pursue faith-in-truth rally together to make their collective voices heard. Many of us are hurting and it is natural to react with a "flee" response. However, if we work together to encourage a Christian community that places the "fruits of the spirit" above political and social gains, we will stand strong again. When we are oppressed, it can be a catalyst for positive radical change. Through oppression hope can grow.

Let's rally together to encourage each other in hope. "So encourage each other and build each other up, just as you are already doing."[18]

Notes:

1 Matthew 7: 15

2 Galatians 5:22

3 Matthew 7: 3

4 Philippians 2

5 Ephesians 4:32

6 Matthew 7

7 Mark 9:35

8 Galatians 5:23

9 Matthew 4:24

10 James 1:27

11 Matthew 15:32

12 Matthew 23:4

13 Mark 12:39

14 Luke 20:46

15 Galatians 3:26

16 Timothy 3:2-8

17 Timothy 3:6-9

18 1 Thessalonians 5:11

Nurture, Nature, Choice

The Biblical Perspective of Jesus in Matthew 19

> *Genesis 1:27 "So God created man in his own image, in the image of God he created him; male and female he created them."*
>
> *Deuteronomy 22: 5 "A woman must not wear men's clothing, nor a man wear women's clothing, for the LORD your God detests anyone who does this."*

For years, these two scripture verses have been thorns in the side of the transgender community. A diligent study of these verses, and a close association with the issues they raise, can lead to a deeper understanding beyond the surface. However, for most in the western church these scriptures raise eyebrows and even deep concerns. (There is a lot going on here, and it will take more then just a few sentences to unpack this.)

You may be surprised to learn that these same verses were discussed and debated in regards to gender identity and issues of social norms even back in the time of Jesus, and apparently before!

On the surface, these verses sound pretty straightforward don't they? But wait, these verses are not stand-a-lone thoughts. As with every other scripture, we should ask, "What is the context? Who is the audience. What about the other verses around them?"

The most damning of the two (as it is applied to the transgender community) is the verse in Deuteronomy 22:5. It is important to note that this verse is sandwiched between many other verses. Some refer to the treatment of found objects; what to do with a lost ox or donkey; gathering of eggs; and safety features for roofing. Some have to do with not mixing things together: two kinds of cloth; two kinds of seeds; and yoking an ox and a donkey together. Another verse refers to the mandate to wear tassels on your clothing. Most of these verses are viewed as very specific to the times back then and not readily applicable today. Even so, it is amazing how some Bible readers peruse these verses in Deuteronomy, picking and choosing for themselves which verse they should follow and which are culturally irrelevant. These verses are treated as if they were a smorgasbord of rules, some we choose while others are harder to stomach.[3]

Regardless, this verse (Deut. 22:5) is often picked out of the group and used to make a case against those who would act outside of cultural norms in terms of dress. This part of Deuteronomy contains a large amount of verses concerning marriage as well. Most of it, in fact, talks about marriage and divorce. Although the verse about wearing clothing of the opposite gender may seem unconnected to the verses concerning marriage, apparently there is a relevant connection that both the Pharisees and Jesus were aware of. Jesus discussed this connection in Matthew 19.

It is obvious from scripture that many of the concerns and issues raised in Old Testament times are outside of our modern experience. However, the topics of marriage, gender, and gender-based social functions are still very much in the news today. The debate on who can be legally married is taking place all over the world. There are a lot of heated discussions around the subject of gender today. Gender roles, marriage, gender identity, and

---

3 Other verses in this passage are today summarily dismissed as no longer culturally relevant. So why is there still so much attention given to the verse in Deuteronomy 22:5? We would see their treatment of women as appalling today. Some of the more alarming verses in Deuteronomy include: "If a man happens to meet a virgin who is not pledged to be married and rapes her and they are discovered, he shall pay the girl's father fifty shekels of silver. He must marry the girl, for he has violated her. He can never divorce her as long as he lives." Also, "If a man happens to meet in a town a virgin pledged to be married and he sleeps with her, you shall take both of them to the gate of that town and stone them to death—the girl because she was in a town and did not scream for help, and the man because he violated another man's wife. You must purge the evil from among you." Those small towns! This was at a time when some men considered women on par with property. Very applicable for today! Seriously, these passages were meant for and relevant to historical Israel. It is not our job to go back in time and pass judgment, nor should their judgments be readily applicable to us today. However, if you dig hard enough there are sound principles at work here, but literally little more. A casual reading of these verses could, and more than likely would, lead to a false conclusion. The Bible is a Historical book as well as one that is inspired. Much of what is written simply recounts what is taking place, and can give us insight into how it was back then. From that understanding, we are able to understand where we are now.

gender-based cultural opportunities were very rigid in the time of Christ, and so questioning them much more controversial back then.

A casual reading of Deuteronomy 22:5 appears straight forward. However, this verse about men wearing women's clothing and women wearing men's clothing may have had more to do with deception in warfare, then much to do with someone's gender identity. Some men pretended to be women to avoid detection as soldiers.

What is clear in the reading is the idea that taking on a role not culturally aligned to one's gender was unacceptable. The divisions of duties in society were along strict the gender lines. (This we will look at later in more detail.)

Marriage, Gender Roles and Gender Identity

A discussion of the issue of gender variance would, in Jesus' day, have included the passages about marriage found in Deuteronomy 22 and 24, as well as the verse in Genesis 1:27. It states,

> *"So God created man in his own image, in the image of God he created him; male and female he created them."*

Again, this looks cut and dry. We are born as we are in the image of God; so don't mess with God's perfect creation.

However, chronologically speaking, a few significant things happen after this event. One of them being the "fall." Man and woman were both turned out of the garden, and sin began to take hold of us. All that has transpired since is off the mark of God's perfect creation. The Bible records our attempts at getting "back to the garden" including genocidal wars on the part of Israel, ridged food preparation laws, and other wonderful ideas such as stoning would-be virgins. I think this illustrates just how far we are living off the mark, and more importantly how impossible it is for the "garden" to be revisited. Even though the attempt may be worthwhile, the reality of what we have created as a result of the "fall" cannot be ignored.

In ancient times your gender and your role in society was rigidly linked. Princes became Kings. Mothers taught daughters to be wives. Carpenters taught their sons the trade. And men and women were to marry, to procreate and raise children. It was assumed that if you were a man you would take a wife (at least one).

In light of this, those who were born without a specific gender or with both genders required a special consideration. Those who did not fully identify with their birth sex or gender and desired not to be in the role of father or mother, husband or wife, presented a real problem.

This "problem" was an issue back then as well as now. Jesus, as part of his teaching in Matthew 19 cites the same two Biblical references that are being cited today. What we would today call the transgender issue was apparently addressed, discussed, and argued with strong opinions back then as well.

It is difficult to know how often Jesus discussed this issue, or what its significance was in the community as a whole. This issue was, at least, important enough to make it into scripture and addressed in the teachings of Jesus.

The Pharisees Set a Trap

In Matthew 19 we find the Pharisees once again approaching Jesus with the intent to trip him up. They ask, "Is it lawful for a man to divorce his wife for any and every reason?"

It is reasonable to suppose that this is not the first conversation they have had with Jesus concerning this issue. The Pharisees are alluding to passages concerning marriage in Deuteronomy 22 that state,

> *"She shall continue to be his wife; he must not divorce her as long as he lives."*

They must of thought this was a trap because this verse does not jell with the scripture in Deuteronomy 24:

> *"When a man takes a wife and marries her, and it happens that she finds no favor in his eyes because he has found some indecency in her, and he writes her a certificate of divorce and puts it in her hand and sends her out from his house..."*

I doubt Jesus was unaware of where they were going with this, but he addresses the issue of male and female as it relates to marriage. Continuing in Matthew 19, Jesus says:

> *"Haven't you read," he replied, "that at the beginning the Creator 'made them male and female, and said, 'For this reason a man will leave his father and mother and be united*

> *to his wife, and the two will become one flesh? So they are no longer two, but one. Therefore what God has joined together, let man not separate."*

He is citing the verse found in Genesis 1:27 which states the condition before the fall. Matthew 19 continues:

> *"Why then," they asked, "did Moses command that a man give his wife a certificate of divorce and send her away?"*

They have him now -- or so they think. Either way Jesus answers they have a ready argument. However Jesus replies in a way that is unexpected and again pushes the limits of their cultural reality. He sees where the Pharisees are going. Matthew 19 continues:

> *Jesus replied, "Moses permitted you to divorce your wives because your hearts were hard. But it was not this way from the beginning. I tell you that anyone who divorces his wife, except for marital unfaithfulness, and marries another woman commits adultery."*

This was unexpected. Jesus addresses the surface issue and closes the door on the issue they were intending to trap him in. He once again addresses the intent of the person instead of their actions. Jesus focuses in on the intent of the relationship and refuses to get caught up in the issue of legality. His answer has an air of authority behind it that has caught even the disciples by surprise. And I can see the Pharisees off to the side wondering at first how to answer this teacher. As they are pondering what to say next, the disciples take up the argument for them. They must have smiled as the disciples joined in, apparently taking the side of the Pharisees. Matthew 19 continues:

> *The disciples said to him, "If this is the situation between a husband and wife, it is better not to marry."*

They knew that Jesus was not in favor of divorce. Prodding Jesus to say he was against divorce was not much of a trap in itself. Besides, how is pointing out scriptures that may contradict each other a trap for Jesus? If this wasn't the ultimate objective of the Pharisees, then what was? In this debate, Jesus found himself on the opposite side to both the Pharisees and the disciples.

Jesus the Radical

Jesus often challenged the notions of cultural, gender and social class lines in his actions and teachings. It is safe to imagine that this sort of teaching did not sit well with the Pharisees. A close look at Jesus' final answer to the question of divorce gives a clear indication as to what the Pharisees had in mind by steering Jesus into the theological neighborhood of marriage, gender roles and gender identity. Jesus could have stayed on the strict issue of divorce by citing other Old Testament laws concerning the appropriate time and place to divorce, but he decides to cut to the chase instead. He addresses the issue of gender identity as it relates to marriage, an issue that rocks the very foundation of who we are as people. It is apparent that the subject of people caught between genders has been raised before, and so Jesus knows where this is going. Jesus exercises his authority as a respected teacher and jumps ahead (like He often does) to the real issue, making a very emphatic statement. He realizes most in his culture, including his disciples, will not be able to understand what He is about to say. Matthew 19 continues:

> *Jesus replied, "Not everyone can accept this word, but only those to whom it has been given. (The ability to understand what he is about to say goes against the current cultural grain and must come through revelation.) For some are eunuchs because they were born that way; others were made that way by men; and others have renounced marriage because of the kingdom of heaven. The one who can accept this should accept it."*

Wow! Nature, nurture, choice. The word eunuch[4] was used to describe those males who were not able to, or apparently unwilling to, marry and raise children in the traditional sense. (The words transgender or inter-

---

4 The oldest available version of Matthew is a translation probably from Aramaic or Hebrew into Greek, and the word used in the Greek translation is eunouchos, from which we get our word eunuch. The word eunouchos comes from eune (bed) and echein (to hold), and most scholars accept that it means "one who guards the bed." But Jesus would not have used the Greek word, since he spoke Aramaic. The Hebrew and Aramaic word for eunuch is saris, an Assyrian loan word that has been interpreted to mean "at the head." an ancient Syriac translation of the Bible used the word mu'omin for eunouchos and saris. Mu'omin means "person of faith" or "person of trust." Theological Dictionary of the New Testament states: The article on the word eunouchos by Johannes Schneider stated that the Greek word appeared in two chapters in the New Testament, and the Hebrew word saris occurred 40 times in the Old Testament (which was underestimated). Moreover, Schneider asserted that many men were called saris in the Old Testament who were not actually eunuchs, by which he meant to say they were not castrated. Schneider also mentioned a discussion in the Talmud concerning differences between born versus man-made eunuchs. The context of nature, nurture and choice was one associated with the word saris which opens up the application to include eunuchs that were not castrated, but chose that life. The application to modern day could easily incorporate many who are transgender. This is by no means a Biblical stretch, but inherent in the lesson application and language.

sexed were not available then, but the word "saris" included those who functioned as eunuchs, or lived outside of their male gender role, even though they had functioning genitalia.*) If the term eunuch referred only to those who had non-functioning genitalia, then why the words, "Not everyone can accept this word, but only those to whom it has been given?" It would not take a special faith to understand that some men had genitals that did not function. For that matter, why discuss eunuchs at all when talking about divorce? These people would not have been married anyway so why drag them into a discussion about marriage? It is obvious that Jesus is making a statement about the male gender role and the validity of living outside of that role. Jesus may have held unpopular or untraditional views concerning male and female gender roles, but why are the Pharisees so interested in getting Jesus to talk about this subject?

The Pharisees were very practiced in the creation of Biblical argument. The hot topic of nature, nurture and choice was one that could be used against Jesus to drive a wedge between him and his disciples. Jesus tried to make others understand his insights but was limited to the understanding and the culture of the day. The Pharisees knew how Jesus felt about this issue and that his radical thoughts were not shared by many.

Jesus is saying that born that way, made that way and chosen to be that way are equally valid reasons for a person to be outside of cultural gender. This by itself is radical. It goes beyond even the current debate of "nature vs nurture." Jesus expands the debate to include "choice." This third possibility of "choice," even today, is the one condition that both sides of the issue agree is invalid. Both sides see "choice" as a deal breaker and the argument has been focused (for at least 2,000 years) on biology vs environment. In response to this, not only does Jesus validate the idea of choice as a reason equal to nature and nurture, but goes on to elevate it above the others with this statement: "...and others have renounced marriage because of the kingdom of heaven." WOW! Even in today's modern society, the idea we can choose a gender role outside of the norm (for ourselves) is very radical and not at all popular. That to "choose" to do so could be for heavenly reasons is very radical indeed. It was this "trap" that the Pharisees wanted him to step in. Rather than fleeing this unpopular opinion, Jesus states his position clearly, and ends with "The one who can accept this should accept it."

Many of his teachings fell on seemingly deaf ears, because those listening had no point of reference to understand what he was saying. Many of Jesus' teachings confused even those closest to him on a regular basis. According to a quick accounting, there are over two dozen references found in the gospels that refer to a "lack of understanding" on the part of those who were listening to the teachings of Jesus. Jesus said to them, "Is this not the reason you are mistaken, that you do not understand the Scriptures or the power of God?"

Next time you are arguing for the rights of the transgender community, remember even Jesus had difficulty convincing someone who did not have the life experience, perspective or insight necessary for understanding.

Jesus accepted those who were honest and truthful about who they were. He allowed for and embraced those who were living outside the cultural gender norms. Think this is the only incident that alludes to gender roles? Read the account of the Last Supper in Mark 14. (I'm surprised to see any reference to gender issues in Scripture considering how uncomfortable this issue makes people.) Mark 14 reads:

> *"On the first day of the Feast of Unleavened Bread, when it was customary to sacrifice the Passover lamb, Jesus' disciples asked him, "Where do you want us to go and make preparations for you to eat the Passover?"*
>
> *So he sent two of his disciples, telling them, "Go into the city, and a man carrying a jar of water will meet you. Follow him. Say to the owner of the house he enters, 'The Teacher asks: Where is my guest room where I may eat the Passover with my disciples?' He will show you a large upper room, furnished and ready. Make preparations for us there."*

Why were the disciples only told to follow a man? Which man? Why say that he was carrying water? What would be the significance of that action? How many men would be drawing water? Not many, for the work of drawing water was that of a woman. The women often would go to draw water and take the opportunity to visit about their days. This was not unlike a beauty parlor experience. However, here was a man in the role of a woman employed by someone who obviously was okay with the gender bending. From the scripture it is reasonable to guess that this was not the homeowner's first encounter with Jesus. This person obviously knew Jesus would be coming by and had already prepared the room for him and his crew. Jesus chose this home to eat the most important meal of his ministry. The home of someone who was coloring outside the gender lines.

Still not convinced? Then let me just say, *"The one who can accept this should accept it."*

Am I Compromising My Faith By Dwelling in God's Grace?

Q: Am I compromising my faith if I explore gender identity issues? Am I making the same mistakes as the Israelites in the Old Testament and the churches in Revelations?

When the call went forth for an uncompromising lifestyle in the Old Testament, even the most well meaning persons fell short. The same was true for the seven Churches in Revelations and those churches Paul wrote to in the New Testament. There are some success stories, but most of what we read are accountings of the failures of God's people. Why record so many failures? Is the Old Testament trying to challenge us to surpass the failed attempts of the Israelites? Is that why these stories are included in the Bible? Do we think we can live our lives in a more righteous way than God's chosen people?

Perhaps questions about righteous actions and godly living are not the most important questions after all, nor the point of these historical accountings. If they aren't, then what is the point of these stories? What does God want us to learn? What is God trying to teach us through the trials of our spiritual forefathers?

Uncompromised Living - Myth or Promise?

Even the most elementary understanding of God's glory and perfection, makes one realize that godly perfection here on Earth is unattainable. God, who knows all things, knows it is impossible for us to live an uncompromised lifestyle. A truly uncompromised life is one that is perfect and flawless. Unfortunately, we do not have the resources to live such a life. Our human nature rejects the commitment it would take to attempt such a monumental undertaking. Our missing the mark of perfection is often referred to in the extreme as "sin." In the church "sin" becomes more than just a word to describe our shortcomings, but is seen as a tangible entity with a personality of its own. Many in the church fear the thought of sin as one might fear the boogieman or the devil. Imperfection then becomes intolerable with eternal punishment as the consequence. This idea has been promoted from many pulpits to keep congregants in line through fear.

Our attempts to understand the life of Christ are filtered through our own prejudices. Therefore, those who think that they can meet God's standards are those who do not know what God's standards are.

We all fall into the trap of projecting our own sensibilities and desires onto what we think the character of God is. But because of our limited understanding of God, the standard we erect is, in essence, no more than a glorified view of self. We cannot help this, for our understanding of life stems only from our own experiences. Most of us know however that our view of God is incomplete. This should compel us to be more open and circumspect when trying to understand the character of God, but unfortunately it sometimes does the opposite. Our lack of knowledge is often rationalized as an unavoidable deficit and so therefore excused. We claim only to be accountable for what we know and assign the label of "mystery" to whatever that other unattainable knowledge might be.

Those who think they can understand the standard of God have deluded themselves and lowered the bar (the standard of God) to a level they can more easily step over. Instead of comparing themselves to God's standards and developing a humble spirit, they measure their success by focusing in on the failure of others. This allows them to puff themselves up with pride in their own accomplishments and demonstrations of measured self-control. They pride themselves on what they haven't done, and point to those who have not achieved their level of piety. The log in their eye is not as important as the speck in their brother's eye. They define for themselves what comprises an uncompromised lifestyle by including those things they desire and exclude those conditions they find reprehensible. This is usually done by grading sins from unforgivable, to unavoidable, to acceptable. Those things they desire, that may very well be sin, they classify as either "acceptable under grace," or an "unavoidable condition of the womb."

Unfortunately, we care what they think.

Tragically, those of us who are singled out as "unclean," often concur with the assessment of those who judge us. We allow them to define for us what an uncompromised or holy life is. We agree with them, and try to live up to their standards. According to them we have two choices; follow them, or burn in hell. They instruct us to earn their idea of heaven, or perish outside the walls of their community.

If you reject their assessment of you as obviously unchristian and unloving, you create a third choice. The third choice is to redefine what an uncompromised lifestyle is for yourself and so lower or re-adjust the bar so you can step over it. Once you determine the height of your righteousness-bar, then the attempt is made to find others who agree with you and will uphold your newfound faith. This new group then searches the scriptures in order to justify their insights. Armed with Biblical redefinitions and newfound awareness, those past spiritual leaders are judged to be legalistic, unloving or just plain ignorant. Eventually we find others who cannot step over "our bar" and so create our own little niche in the erroneous spiritual smorgasbord of "wrong and right" as we vilify them and so, by contrast justify ourselves. By this, we have become the legalist, and have entered into the same condemnation as those who previously spurned us.

The fault of the legalist is not that they have taken and raised the bar too high, but that they have blinded themselves to their own sins and shortcomings and lowered the bar. We must leave the bar (the measure of righteousness) where it is. Even though we know the bar can never be reached. This is the point of trying to live the uncompromised life: we can't do it!

This may sound rather bleak, but our human condition compared to God's glory is rather bleak. To try and live up to Gods' standards is hopeless. So enters grace.

A Godly Perspective

Obviously, the scriptures are not there to define for us "who is better than whom." The argument as to who will be greater in the kingdom of heaven, started by Christ's own disciples, continues today. Comparisons with each other only lead to self condemnation or self glorification that hamper a true understanding of what it means to be righteous. We cannot, through the law or our accomplishments, perfect the work of Christ beyond his free gift of grace. It is perfect as it is, and God requires little or nothing on our part to redeem us. Christ lived a flawless life, but even those who followed him did not understand what he was saying. Many, because of their prejudice, saw his life as blasphemous. Even his miraculous actions were questioned. His life was misunderstood then, and is still misunderstood today. The message of the gospels is the message of a grace we can barely understand. The accomplishment of the cross pierces our sinful nature in a way that is beyond comprehension. To gain any true knowledge of grace is to understand just how unfathomable it really is.

Is God mocking us?

In the Old Testament God mandates that we attempt to live a "sin-free" life with dire consequences for those who do not comply, knowing full well that we are doomed to fail.

This idea of futility goes against our human nature and our inbred idea of fairness. When we begin a task, we must have some sort of reasonable expectation of success. Otherwise we deem the attempt a futile one. If you knew a task was doomed for failure from the start, and that there was absolutely no chance of success, would you begin the task anyway? Our human brains must have a clear idea of what a righteous life is, so we emulate people around us and try and mimic those things they do, or don't do. This we call righteousness. (This is usually a glorified form of self). We doubt that God would ask us to try and attempt a standard so high that even the attempt itself would even be a sin. But that is exactly what we are being asked to do.

God has asked us to begin a task that is impossible to complete. God asks us to attempt something that is futile and confusing in its directions. Why? Because the main point of the Old Testament and the New Testament was to point to the grace bought by the sacrifice of Jesus. Yet we still feel the need to claim some sort of righteousness for ourselves. We still need to justify our actions. We still need to feel good about our choices and somehow exalt them up to a level that is beyond debate, beyond question.

God knows we will fail. Yet we still try, thinking that we can somehow measure up. We still hope to somehow control our destiny by purchasing what we cannot possibly earn.

So what would God have us do?

It isn't until we say with Paul, "I am the worst of all sinners!" that we truly begin a journey, not towards refinement of self-righteousness and the law, but towards God. We do not change our hearts!! God does!!

"Why do you ask, "Why did you create me like this? You cannot change the color of one hair on your head..."

We learn from the Israelites, not how to do it better or different, but we learn from them that the attempt is futile if your objective is to succeed. We should not look at the law as a mandate, but as a road map. We should try to understand that all of our attempts at righteousness are no more than filthy rags and trust that God is real and ultimately in control.

Our focus should be on our relationship with God and we should embrace the fact that it is only through grace that we have an audience before the throne. Grace tells us, "I will remove your sin from you, as far as the earth is from the sky so shall I remove your sin." Under grace, the issue of sin in our lives is reduced to a spiritual sidebar and not the main focus of what it means to be a follower of Christ. The law, works and sin all declare us dead to God. Only grace declares us redeemed.

The God of grace is loving and accepting. "While we were yet sinners, Christ died for us." God is loving, but remains true to God's holy character.

Q: If God has a problem with LGBTQI+ people, then how can we fellowship with them? Isn't being transgender a sin? I listen to my brothers and sisters in Christ telling me that any LGBTQI+ person cannot be a Christian as long as they live as they do. If a long time Christian comes out as LGBTQI+ then perhaps they were never saved in the first place.

A: That question could also be asked in reverse. Is being LGBTQI+ a sinless, perfect state? Obviously, the answer to that question is the same for any life lived — *obviously "no."* Every life-style is short of godly-perfection since there is always a human element attached. So if the question, "Are lesbian, gay, bisexual, transgender or queer people short of godly perfection" then yes they are, just like everyone else. It is clear from scripture that EVERY person and lifestyle falls short of perfection and therefore is, by definition, sinful. That said, those who ask these sorts of questions or have these sorts of sin-focused concerns, demonstrate an infantile understanding of what sin is, especially in the light of grace.

Our understanding of sin needs to be more evolved and aligned more closely to the Apostle Paul who declared himself, "the worst of all sinners." Paul understood that we mistakenly try to justify our actions and lifestyles by recoursing Biblical law, when the purpose of the law is to point us to grace. He wrote about this in Romans 3:19-24:

> *"Now we know that whatever the Law says, it speaks to those who are under the Law, so that every mouth may be closed and all the world may become accountable to God; because by the works of the Law no flesh will be justified in His sight; for through the Law comes the knowledge of sin. But now apart from the Law the righteousness of God has been manifested, being witnessed by the Law and the Prophets, even the righteousness of God through faith in Jesus Christ for all those who believe; for there is no distinction; for all have sinned and fall short of the glory of God, being justified as a gift by His grace through the redemption which is in Christ Jesus...*

You can argue the fine points of the issue and try and justify through a re-working of the scriptures, but an honest look at all these lifestyles shows them to be short of godliness. But then we come back to the real question; what is a godly lifestyle?

Any person who has lived more than a few years with Christ knows how sinful and ungodly any of our lifestyles are. If you do not see your lifestyle as sinful, then you are aligned with the Pharisees, and I hope God will not leave you in this wretched state. *"It would be better if you had a millstone tied around your neck and you were cast into the sea."* (Luke 17:2)

However, since we are saved by grace, then what is the point of weeding out sinners from among us? Could any one of us stand up to honest scrutiny? We are saved into a relationship and it will be GOD who will judge them (and us), and turn their hearts (and ours) when it is necessary. "If we judge them, we judge ourselves for we practice the same things!" Jesus said, *"Even if you think such a thing, you are guilty..."* Jesus raised the bar beyond the reach of everyone. Many do not believe this, because they do not see their own sin. They have little or no concept of the glory of God and so have settled for a form of God that is more comfortable.

You may say, "Okay, I agree with that, but doesn't God call us to live righteously anyway?"

Yes, but it is the righteousness of Christ that we live in, not our own righteousness. As it reads in Ephesians 2:8-10: *"For by grace you have been saved through faith; and that not of yourselves, it is the gift of God; not as a result of works, so that no one may boast. For we are God's workmanship, created in Christ Jesus for good works, which God prepared beforehand so that we would walk in them."*

We were saved from the power of sin to separate us from God, but not from our sinful actions. We were saved from many of the consequences of our poor choices, but not from our free will. Salvation inspires a radical change of heart and is forever life changing. Being saved usually goes hand-in-hand with a spiritual awakening. The joy of this change often compels us to change things in our lives. When we are saved, we often lose interest in certain (sinful) actions that we previously held onto, but do not confuse that "cleansing" with salvation. We still fall short of God's glory. We can make no claim that supersedes or invalidates the ongoing work of grace.

Q: Am I denying God's will, by not renouncing my transgender nature? How can I convince someone that I'm not compromising my faith?

A: Yes, it is true that you are settling for a lifestyle that is less than godly perfection, but you are also being realistic and honest about who you are. That said, grace and a voluntary acceptance of your own shortcomings will deflate the self-condemnation fueling this question. Honestly accepting yourself is more important to God than any attempt on your part to circumvent grace. For how could we sinful creatures ever think we, through our own effort, ever abide in God's perfect will? We are powerless to know it, and to seek it is an impossible task. However, the good news is that grace is not powerless. Grace covers all. God redeems our seemingly futile attempts and creates something far more glorious than we could have imagined. Jesus did miracles on the Sabbath which was forbidden. But it was not reckoned to him as sin because he understood the essence of the scriptures.

As God left the thorn in the flesh in the Apostle Paul, God has not changed my transgender nature. If this is a weakness, then may God use that weakness. For when I am weak, I can take no credit for the good God can do through me.

You ask if your CDing or T-nature is a sinful state? You could argue that either way. If those are the types of questions burning in your heart, then your compass is not pointing true north. God loves you as you are. That should be your compass.

For me, God has allowed my trans nature to remain so that I can relate and have more empathy for others and share God's love. Do I take my freedom in Christ to CD as a mandate from God? Is God telling me that others, like myself, are justified in doing whatever they please? No, my freedom in Christ is not a call to condemn or condone the actions of others.

In the second part of your question about "convincing others" perhaps you can show that you are not compromising by telling them the truth about your spiritual walk. Be candid about what God is doing in your life. Let them know about your journey and struggles. Truth provides clarity and connection.

To answer their concerns directly: I would not call it a compromise, but rather a realistic evaluation of where you are currently, and of your utter dependence on grace.

Ask yourself this, "Have you felt a deep affection for those in the transgender community who are being oppressed, who do not have the resources to improve their lives? If you have empathized with them, and felt their pain, then that is the heart of God expressing itself in and through you.

Take time with God to focus on the good you can do and do not let your shortcomings or "sin nature" define you. A focus on sin can be a debilitating hindrance. We think that it is our sinful actions that separate us from God, but that is not the case. Jesus has demonstrated that you have access to God even in your flawed state. You might only see the glory of God dimly now, but you can still join with God's heart and reach out to those in need. When you demonstrate, as Jesus did, the fruits of the spirit in your life you align yourself with, and draw closer to, God

I know that if God had deleted my transgender nature, I would have become like those who throw stones. I am the person that God wants me to be. God works with and through me — an imperfect creature relying on grace.

I realize that the grace I count on will appear as a compromise to some. And yes, I could be wrong in my assessment of the situation, but I would rather follow Christ and his example of love than to slide into a legalistic mindset of condemnation and despair. I do not fear being wrong and my failings do not define me — that is grace.

Because of my arrogance, it might take wallowing a bit in the mud to remind me how filthy I am. When I am weak, God is stronger.

To sum up, do not defend your position for it is indefensible and the attempt will only cause further division. Be resolved in your choice.

As you follow the path of Christ try and avoid spiritual road-rage. Do not enter into a discussion with someone who only wants to argue and has no interest in an honest dialogue aimed at discovering truth.

Or you can simply echo the words of Paul, "God does not judge me (so as to change), so I do not judge myself, and so you don't judge me."

Do Your Clothes Fit?

What is your motive for dressing up in clothing of the 'opposite' gender?

Feeling comfortable in one's clothing is almost the same as feeling comfortable in one's own skin. Are we somehow sinning if we hate the way we look, or are repulsed by our appearance? Are we rejecting a fundamental gift of God? Are we second-guessing the Creator and calling into question the creative process as it pertains to us?

There are verses in the Bible that talk about our bodies being the temple of God. One is found in 1 Corinthians 3:16:

> *"Don't you know that you yourselves are God's temple and that God's Spirit lives in you? If anyone destroys God's temple, God will destroy him; for God's temple is sacred, and you are that temple."*

We are to cherish that which God has given to us. The Bible also speaks of certain facts concerning our bodies:

> *"...no one ever hated his own body, but he feeds and cares for it..." Ephesians 5:29*

These may sound like admonishments to keep us in peak physical condition, and not allow ourselves to be maimed. However, as with many scriptures, this is not the whole truth. If the command were a rigid, "Do not alter, nor have harm caused to your being, because you should at all times glorify God by the presentation of a healthy body," then Christ would have been at fault when he allowed himself to be crucified. Obviously, there are other considerations that may be more important.

Wearing clothing of the "opposite gender" is an attempt to alter one's self-perception. When doing so, the image in the mirror can provide a sense of normalcy. Is making yourself over in this fashion against the fundamental will of God? Should the practice of cross-dressing (CDing) in light of these scriptures be questioned? It is always important to check our motives and be deliberate in what we do.

So what is the motive? Is it to flee from God's creation, or is it to move towards acceptance of it? Perhaps it is a bit of both.

For most who cross-dress, their CDing sessions are like therapy. It is a way to connect with the part of yourself that was previously squelched. In a sense, one image is rejected in favor of the other. But in another sense, this activity can be useful to help recapture a sense of balance. The pendulum swings in both directions, and for many years perhaps it was pushed too far in one direction. So, if it now goes too far the other way, it is with the hope it will eventually swing back towards the middle at some point. There is some damage control that needs to be addressed. God understands this and grace covers this process.

It is not just a matter of accepting who we are on the outside; the real struggle is trying to accept who we are on the inside. If we can do this, then what we accomplished will last, even after the make-up is sponged off, and the wig is back in its box.

Where do these feelings of body-loathing come from? What can be done about them? Can we, through sheer will, stop feeling a certain way? Perhaps the answer again is both "yes" and "no."

"No" in that it is nearly impossible to rewind the tape of our life and begin over again. We cannot avoid altogether the destructive narrow society in which we have been raised. We are stuck with our notions of beauty and gender roles, ingrained in us since birth. Yet, the answer can also be "yes", in that we can honestly face our shortcomings. It is because we are saved by grace, and that God wishes for us to know the truth about ourselves that we can come to grips with who we are, and where God wants us to go.

There have been times in our lives when we nourished our flesh, and cared for it. There have been times when we saw ourselves as the temple of God. Perhaps only when we were young, but those times did exist. The image we embraced as a child (a very young child) was the truth of who we are. We need to remember that truth.

So how do we get some of this healthy, godly perspective back?

First by recognizing that we are purposefully created. It may not "feel" that way, but we can begin to intellectually agree with the precept. The second is to begin the process of chipping away at the hard bitter scales of self-loathing that now cover the body. Try to reverse some of the emotional damage that has been done. Clothing apparently can be an easy way to start.

I heard a song on the radio yesterday. One of the verses went something like, "When all of your clothes feel like somebody's old throw-a-ways..."

That sums it up fairly well. As we get older our clothes may not fit as well as they once did. Our bodies and minds change and so should our clothing to reflect that change. Don't always wait until your clothes wear out. Perhaps when you were young you wore hand-me-downs. Chances are they never really felt right. Once new, these clothes had now been well worn. A once bright orange T-shirt is now a dim peach color. Pulling it over your head, you feel it scratch along your skin and pinch under your arms. The whole shirt was twisted and stretched to fit someone else's body, not yours. The real you is being usurped and invalidated with a covering not reflective of your identity.

Christmas presents were always looked forward to. I must have been 8-years-old this particular Christmas. A brightly wrapped box lay under the tree in expectation of my wide-eyed discovery. Of course clothing was not usually on my wish list, but as long as it wasn't underwear or socks, I didn't mind too much. This particular package's turn had arrived. I sat on the floor with my legs crossed with the box on my lap. Tearing open one end, I pulled the box out from underneath its wrapper. I broke the tape that held on the lid. Lifting up one side, I reached in to see if I could guess what it was. My fingers told me it was rough. Good. It wasn't underwear, I thought, at least I sincerely hoped not.

I started to form some guesses. A new jacket? Perhaps a shirt? Maybe a new pair of jeans; the kind that would "squeak" as you walked down the halls at school. The feel of something new was always appreciated. Finally, I pulled the new treasure out from under its lid. It was pants. Purple ones. I was flabbergasted. Purple pants? She had bought purple pants? I then flashed back on a moment, a few months before, when my mother had asked me what my favorite color was. I had indeed told her it was purple. So that Christmas I received one pair of pants, one shirt, a jacket and socks...all purple. Since then, whenever anyone inquires as to my favorite color, I always answer black - it's safer.

A couple of years ago I was out shopping, needing to purchase some replacement items, and I began to realize that I was still under the influence of the fashion sense of my older brother and my mother. I gravitated towards the familiar, no matter how cold it left me inside. I realized that in many ways, my mother was still dressing me. Being "thrifty" I became aware that almost none of the items I wore were purchased by me. Most of my wardrobe was comprised of Christmas and birthday gifts, sporting event give-a-ways, hand-me-ups and downs, task-specific items, and yes, still even some thrift store purchases.

Since then, I have tried to make a conscious effort to actually shop for some clothing that speaks of who I am. What I really want to do is find an expression that more closely resembles how I feel inside. With all the choices available, I should be successful.

If you have not been clothes shopping for awhile, perhaps it is time. Purchase something that you like, and is comfortable. You may be surprised by how it makes you feel. You may not feel like you deserve it, but you might just need it.

Is Cross-dressing A Sin?

A Perspective on Grace

This article is in response to an question LITC received. For this person, the question of sin is extremely important. The response given is aligned with that concern. The issue of sin is dealt with directly so that those who also worry about sin can hopefully find a path forward.

> Q: *I feel awful about my cross-dressing. Am I in hopeless sin when I cross-dress?*

For those of you who have beaten yourself up for years trying to fight your transgender nature, may I offer some hope.

You may have spent decades fighting your transgender nature. Perhaps you grew up believing it to be evil (sin). Your cross-dressing (CDing) was usually done in secret and was combined with experiences you would rather not talk about. I have heard a lot of discussion on both sides of the issue. Is CDing wrong or right - sin or not? My angle on this is a little unusual.

I really do not know if CDing can be considered a sin or not. Advocates on both sides of this issue offer compelling arguments. I am interested in the debate, but not overly concerned about its resolution. In either case, a definitive answer appears to be elusive.

In regards to importance, the issue of "sin" takes a backseat to good mental health and the exploration of who we are as God's children. The God of love who desires for us to be happy and whole and has bestowed grace on us to do so. God is more loving and more tolerant with us than we could ever be with each other. We apparently are more interested in what sin is than who God is.

However, since this is an important question to so many, let's unpack it.

The issue of sin and CDing may be a lightning rod for a much larger issue. CDing was the "thorn" God used to deflate my spiritual ego. This spiritual discomfort caused me to ask two questions: "What is the nature of sin?" -*and*- "At what point does an action become sin?"

In Matthew 5:27, Jesus says we sin even in our thoughts. This, of course, leaves little hope for any of us who wish to be sin-free. In fact, whenever Christ was asked to declare something as sinful, he always presented a larger definition that included those asking the question. Take, for example, the story of the woman caught in adultery. (John 8:3) The Pharisees brought a woman before Jesus and wanted his approval to stone her to death. He acknowledged the woman's sin, but went on to say, *"...He who is without sin cast the first stone."* Even though some came to the scene with rocks already in hand, no one threw a stone, for each of them knew, they too, had sins.

Why would Jesus do this? Why expand the parameters of sin? Because, Christ purposed to make the "narrow way" to God even more narrow, so we would have no option but to lean on the grace he was to purchase on the cross. As he says in John 14:6:

> *"I am the way the truth and the life; no one comes to the Father, but through me."*

The message of the gospel of grace is not one of "trying to do good." Christ did not die to remove sin from our lives, but to remove sin's power to control us. For the power of sin comes from this trap: whether we are fleeing sin, or embracing it, sin still has power over us. Sin wants to dictate our day-to-day agendas.

I used to feel that this emphatically stated "path to God only through Jesus" sounded rather restrictive. However, my perspective changed when I began to understand how Jesus' death on the cross altered forever the power that sin had over us in a way that is unparalleled in human history.

Christ came to set us free, completely free, from the power of sin. As a child of God, the righteousness we have adopted is the righteousness of Christ. Therefore we should no longer be bound by the agenda that sin would have us follow.

Christ recognized the sin of adultery, and the sin of all those present, but dispensed grace in his dealings with the woman and encouraged her. He says to us, *"Follow me, for my load is easy and my burden is light."* He says to us, I want to be your agenda. I will change your heart as I see fit. I will be your guide, focus on me. We are now free to explore, as our Savior leads, because we are under the GRACE of God.

Am I saying that sin is irrelevant? On the surface it may appear so, but actually it is just the opposite! Sin permeates everything that we do. Separating it out is a winnowing process that takes a lifetime. Trying to determine what is sin is difficult because often those actions our culture has decreed as “obvious sin” are not. On the other hand, some things that our society says are legal, and holds up as worthwhile goals, are in fact sin. Accepting my transgender nature, and God’s grace, has taught me that I am more sinful, not less.

Choosing one particular sin to focus on can have harmful consequences. The danger in vilifying one aspect of our human nature, is that we then, by contrast, tend to justify the rest of what we do. We start to believe that we can somehow earn righteousness if we “just get this one area under control.”

In Matthew chapter 19, a rich young ruler comes to Jesus and asks: *“Teacher, what good thing shall I do that I may obtain eternal life?”* Jesus answers with, *“Why are you asking me about what is good? There is only One who is good...”* He then speaks to the young man about keeping the commandments, and the young man declares he has kept them all. So Jesus gives him another, *“...sell your possessions and give to the poor... come and follow me.”* The young man goes away grieved because he is very rich. Jesus remarks to the disciples present, *“...it is easier for a camel to go through the eye of a needle, than for a rich man to enter the kingdom of God.”*

In Jesus’ day, just as in our day, wealth was viewed as a blessing from God. So when the disciples heard this they were perplexed and asked, *“Then who can be saved?”* I love Jesus’ reply, *“With men this is impossible, but with God all things are possible.”* The point of this exchange was not that wealth is bad, but that there is no “good thing” you can do to enter into Heaven. Why is this important to the transgender believer? Because we are faced with our own human frailty day by day and have the choice to either accept the grace that our Lord freely offers, or drive ourselves crazy trying to do the “right thing” to obtain God’s favor and eternal salvation. What Jesus says to his disciples he says to you, “With man it is impossible, but with God all things are possible.”

Admitting we need God and letting go of our pursuit of self-righteousness is a good place to be spiritually. Our relationship with God should not be linked to our performance. A healthy relationship with our creator is one where we simply fall on our face (give up worrying and fretting), cling to our Savior, and asking God to have mercy on us sinners. God will not judge you but accept you with open arms. With this attitude you can experience the promise:

> *"I will never desert you, nor will I ever forsake you." (Hebrews 13:5)*

If you are struggling, if your pillow is wet with the tears of self-condemnation, my advice to you is "let it all go." Die to your self-righteousness and be reborn with the understanding that you are a redeemed creation and that your life is Christ's and not your own.

God really does desire to give his children good gifts. Trust him and enjoy the ride!

Is Wearing Panties a Sin?

For the conservative Christian the topic of sin comes up frequently. Actions are defined as either sinful or okay. The sin question is often critical to our more conservative readers. We hope this answer will address some of those concerns.

Q: "Although no scripture verse speaks to this directly, is wearing female undergarments underneath your male clothing a sin?"

I think it is a matter of degrees. We live our lives the best we can with what God has given us. If a pair of panties gets you through the day, then maybe that is better than being in a perpetual funk or yelling at everyone because of your ongoing emotional frustration.

We are quick to take a pill in order to relieve stress or depression without any thought of it being sinful. You could look at CDing (cross-dressing) as a way to relieve stress and as a sort of therapy. But for many the question remains: "Is it a sin?"

I think it can be. However, it is really a question of your motives. A "clear conscious" could be a gauge. But I'm not sure how "clear" you would need your conscience to be in order to validate or normalize the action of cross-dressing if you are perpetually conflicted.

My pastor once asked if a person who cross-dresses is making an "uneasy truce with the devil." He was wondering if a person who stopped struggling was giving up the "fight for holiness" and settling instead for second best.

Wasn't God big enough to cure all or struggles? I understood his concern, but I think that question has some serious flaws in its assumptions. One assumption is that a Christian life is functionally sin-free. Another misconception is that sin is somehow "tacked onto" our being and therefore not part of our nature. A third assumption would be that God's chief purpose is to clean us up so that we may be presentable.

There may be some truth in all these assumptions, but because of our limited human experience and understanding the application of these truths can be both dangerous and harmful. The real question we should be asking is "What is the nature of sin and grace?" If we can understand that, then defining specific sins is secondary to our relationship with Christ.

I know that from the day we accept Christ (especially those brought up in the Christian church), we are indoctrinated with the idea that we must be sin-free. In order to strive for this, we are given life examples to emulate (moral heroes to follow). The problem is that these heroes (Biblical or otherwise) are only human and fall far short of God's holiness. In fact, the standard for a completely righteous life is beyond our grasp. This understanding of our sin nature was not meant to cause eternal despair, but rather to encourage us to seek utter dependence on God's grace and forgiveness. However, the concept of grace is something we cannot fully comprehend, for we have no earthly equivalent. God's grace and forgiveness is as far beyond our understanding as God's Holiness is beyond our reach. (Colossians 1:13-14 / John 16:7-16)

In trying to flesh out the grace of God, we tend to use a glorified version of our best selves in guessing God's responses. Because our mirror is dim, we sometimes mistakenly expect God's response to be similar to our own. In response to our sin or failure, we may imagine God saying, "I forgive you, but don't do it again...or else."

We do not understand the goals of God, nor do we comprehend the purpose of our own journey. We try to please or appease God through what we would consider righteous acts. So instead of pursuing and embracing the full spectrum of grace, we set small goals for ourselves with the thought, "If only I could change this about myself, then I would be righteous." (At least that was my thought.) (2 Corinthians 12:9)

Perhaps you believe only one or two things in your life need changing. Or maybe you have a very long list of items you need to work on. No matter how long the list is, it will never be long enough if you desire perfection.

Our imagined righteous standard (the level to which we aspire) will still be far short of God's infinitely higher standard. I suppose what I am saying is, even if our conscious is "clear" in regards to our actions, perhaps it is only clear because we have lowered the standard of God to align with our personal comfort zone. God is once again recreated in our image. God is less powerful, less godly, less tolerant.

The flip side of that coin is just as bad (perhaps even worse). It is the failure of the Pharisees.

They conquered their perceived sin, or abstained from it through sheer willpower. They took pride in the fact that all of the items on their list were checked off. They sought after righteousness as though it could actually be grasped. They thought that there was a certain lifestyle or set of actions (or inactions) that by themselves would be pleasing to God. This righteousness is a form or self-righteousness and in fact is more displeasing to God than those who understand and see their own sin or faults. Hence the reasons for all the run-ins with Jesus. Jesus' strongest words were for those who asked questions like, "Is it wrong to...?" (Matthew 19:3 / Matthew 15:1-2 / Matthew 9:11)

There is nothing wrong with asking "real questions." A real question is one that is open to a truthful answer and not just a confirmation of a presupposition. The question, "is something a sin?" might seem like a reasonable one. However, isn't it true we usually already know the answer before we ask that question? When we ask that question, are we just trying to find a different answer that will be easier for us to live with? Why do we do that? Perhaps it is because we are uncomfortable with grace. To admit we have sin would be to admit we need grace and that would put us totally at the mercy of God.

We feel the need to have some control over our existence (the earthly and eternal). Since we cannot meet our assumed godly standard, we end up either rejecting God altogether, or lowing the standard to make it more attainable. Both actions separate us from the reality of grace and from God. This is the real power of sin; to create a situation that separates us from God.

Four ways that sin causes us to reject God come to mind.

The first is caused by repeated failures in our fight against sin. Through frustration, we may consciously reject God as a hard, unloving taskmaster who has no real interest in us. Perhaps we feel this way because our load seems too heavy. Perhaps we have sought deliverance through prayers, but our petitions go unanswered. Perhaps we have been beaten down by a series of life-events out of our control. Whatever the cause, the result is that our focus is on ourselves and our sins, not where it should be - on God and grace. Sin and guilt forces a wedge between us and grace. We feel as though God's grace could never apply to us because of our unworthiness. The fact is, God's grace applies to us because we are unworthy. (Matthew 9:11-13 / Romans 5:19)

The second way sin causes a division between us and God is when we lower the standards of God to a level that we can attain. Like the Pharisees, we replace the holiness of God with an adherence to cultural norms or a shared sense of moral values. This leads to a rating system of sin. We determine that some sins are worse than others. Some (as we see them) minor sins everyone within our chosen group may commit, so these are OK. We then choose other sins that only a small percentage of our population struggle with, and avoidance of these sins becomes our litmus test for righteousness. Those poor unfortunate souls who struggle with these "pet sins" become our new favorite projects. We work hard on removing the splinters from their eyes, so that they will become more like us. Our focus is on their sin, not grace. As a result, we cease to pursue God's holiness at all and tragically develop a glorified image of ourselves in His place. The pursuit of righteousness has turned into intolerant self-righteousness. We have embraced the song rather than the singer. (Matthew 23:24-29 / Matthew 7:2-5)

The third is much like the second in that we lower the standards of God to a level we feel more comfortable with. However, in this third scenario we declare certain sins not to be sin any longer. Sin becomes subjective. We surround ourselves with people of like mind and embrace a twisted form of grace that does not include a declaration of our own depravity. We cease to take responsibility for our actions using expressions like, "I was made this way." In fact we may go so far as to make our "sin" part of our letterhead. ie: "The First Church of the Filthy Rich" or "Criminals for Christ." Sin has control over us in that the pursuit of justification is more important than the pursuit of the character of Christ. The fact that "we cannot help ourselves" does not automatically make it right to indulge. We need to accept the truth of our sin nature. (Matthew 23:13-15 / Matthew 24:4-5)

The fourth is to wallow in guilt where we are trapped in that place of repeated attempts to "please" God through our actions. We cry out from the depths, unable to find release from our sin nature, but convinced that this place of anxiety and self-condemnation is where we should be. After all, aren't we more pious when we are depressed? We cling like a codependent to a stone image of God. We take the thorn of sin embedded in our skin, and twist it to remind us of just how unworthy we really are. We spend much of our time fighting our "sin" convinced that this is our plight. Ironically, the truth is we are unworthy, but it is only part of the truth. The greater truth is that we are redeemed. Guilt somehow makes us forget that. Even so, we still have a desire to pursue God, but our accuser never ceases day and night to remind us of our unworthiness. Sin has us trapped in an endless circle of defeat, short-lived victory, and purging. (Galatians 3:3-5 / Galatians 3:21-24)

All four scenarios miss the real point of what Jesus accomplished on the cross. Which is this: Grace is the only option for those who want to draw near to God.

I think the real power of sin in our lives comes from setting our daily agenda through guilt. Our performance should not be the measure of the reality of our faith, but sin would have us believe it to be so. If we defeat (for a season) sin through struggle, we are in danger of becoming like the Pharisees. If we fail in that struggle, we may fall under self-condemnation and adopt an attitude of separation from God. Whether we win or lose, sin has set our agenda. Our focus is mistakenly on ourselves and our actions. It no longer becomes a matter of what we should do, but what we should not do. The fight against sin has caused us to take our eyes off of God's calling for us. Don't be a slave to the agenda of sin. Admit you will never be good enough and embrace instead the free gift of grace. Only in this way will you enter into a thankful, living, loving relationship with God. (Galatians 2:19-21)

A truly positive godly life comes from admitting our sin and accepting grace as sufficient. God was not taunting the Apostle Paul when he said "...my grace is sufficient." God loves you as you are. You are redeemed just as you are. There is nothing left but to accept forgiveness and grace. You are God's child. Stop condemning yourself. God does not. (Galatians 4:4-7 / 2 Corinthians 12:9)

Conclusion:

The fabric of your life was created from many different threads. Know and admit that everything you do is not perfect. Every thread is tainted and misses the mark (sin). You are now and always will be a someone saved only by grace. Rejoice in what God has done and cling to God. Just be thankful and do not condemn yourself, because God does not condemn you. You don't have to pay God back. (Romans 3:9-23 / Romans 6:23) In the light of God's astounding grace, all our righteousness and positive works are no better than filthy rags (sin). Jesus set us free from the power of sin. He has freed us up to follow him without guilt and without worry. Give up worrying about "sin" and just accept God's grace, no strings attached. Your relationship with God and those around you should be your principle focus. Don't be distracted from that pursuit. (Galatians 5:1 / Romans 5:1-2)

PS: Oh, I almost forgot. Wearing panties - is it sinful? For those of you who MUST have concrete guidelines: The light colored pink ones are doubtful and perhaps not okay, but the powdered blue ones are fine. Black or white are okay, but not floral patterns. Silky ones are okay as long as they are not a cotton/wool blend, but made from a single type of cloth. Tassels are a plus. But you already knew that, didn't you? Personally, I just try and match my socks. (Kidding of course!)

Legalism and Indulgence

When Is Enough, Enough?

Q: *Aren't the laws of God there for us to vigorously uphold? Isn't it safer to err on the side of legalism?*

I could call this article: "Something funny happened to me on the way to the truth."

I was legalistic when I was younger. Perhaps it was because legalism is easier to understand. Legalism offers a set of structured rules and behavioral guidelines that promise clearly defined compelling rewards. However, in seeking the truth we will eventually discover that legalism uses the tools of fear and guilt to promote a false sense of self.

Legalism, at best, is just a stepping stone to understanding our need for grace. It is, at worst, a road-block that keeps us from pursuing a love-based relationship with our Lord and an honest understanding of who we are. To be bound to legalism is to be bound to a false god created by a minority that filters their understanding through a culture that has an incomplete understanding of who they are before God. Legalism serves not those under its control, but rather the few who try and exercise that control. It robs ALL involved of their humanity and their dignity. It supplants God with an icon engraved with a list of rules. These rules are carefully constructed to condemn anyone outside of their tolerance and to justify their personal preferences.

Legalism, in fact, does exactly the opposite of what it intends. It pushes people away from God. It widens the chasm between God and us by nullifying grace. It holds onto a small amount of truth and declares other revelations irrelevant. It hopes to create a sense of righteousness, but instead creates only a sense of self-righteousness. It excludes those who do not agree and refuses to be moved on any issue. If you want to know the truth about where your church falls short, read the passages in your Bible that are not highlighted.

Understanding the Truth Beyond Legalism

Holding our assumed truths "loosely" is an important attitude if we want to discern between what is real and what is false. The truth is best understood as truth when we make ourselves vulnerable to being wrong.

In order to discover the truth, we must embrace our faults. I must recognize my faults as unhealthy choices for me, and try not to justify them. My faults can include my behavior, my desires, my repulsions, and my thoughts. To discover the truth is to discover a way of life that transcends our presuppositions. The truth can move you beyond legalism and fear - into a place that promotes love and grace.

In the spirit of truth let us take an honest look at 1 Corinthians, chapter six. Paul is addressing the church on the subject of lawsuits. Some of the church members were bringing lawsuits against each other before magistrates that were not Christians and so were using a set of rules and guidelines that were not based on a relationship with God. In verses 1 and 2, Paul was telling them to avoid being judged by the world or under a system that wasn't constructed by God. As we know, God's system is one based on redemption, resurrection, and on grace.

Paul puts our standing before God (as Christians) into perspective by saying, "Do you not know that we shall judge angels?" 1 Corinthians 6: 3

Why does Paul say that we shall judge angels? Of course there are two basic kinds of angels, those who worship God and those fallen angels who are demons. God has already judged the latter. So in what sense do we judge angels? I am not sure. But I do know that Paul raises the point for the purpose of contrast. He is illustrating the fact that we do not need the world's list of do's and don'ts to determine what is right. Paul also says that we should be wary when we put ourselves under the judgment of the world. In other words, we who have been given the authority through the death and resurrection of Christ, to judge even the angels in his name, have chosen in many ways to be judged by the world instead. If we ignore our relationship with God through grace and embrace either legalism and/or the construct of the world, we fall short of truth. When we rely on standards that do not reflect a real relationship with God, we condemn ourselves in our pursuit of the truth.

Paul then talks specifically about the brethren taking other brethren into court. He calls the action itself a defeat. To demand your own rights over those of your brethren is already a defeat for you. Paul says that it is better to be wronged or defrauded than to be in that situation.

Then Paul goes and does something that Christ often did. He expands the definition to include all those who are reading the scripture. Paul says that if we think about it, we have to admit that we are also wrong and have defrauded others as well. All of us are included in this accounting. This goes back to the idea that if we judge others, we judge ourselves.

Paul then hones his point finer. He begins to define some specific ways that separate us from God. Paul writes, "Do you not know that the unrighteous shall not inherit the kingdom of God? Do not be deceived; neither fornicators, nor idolaters, nor adulterers, nor effeminate by perversion, nor homosexuals, nor thieves, nor the covetous (most everyone in the US), nor drunkards, nor revilers, nor swindlers shall inherit the kingdom of God."

This is not an inclusive list by any means, although an honest person will see themselves in at least one of these descriptions. Even so, Paul is not declaring to those who do not find themselves on this list to be "off the hook." This list was chosen not to edify those who think they are not on the list, but rather to isolate specific types of behavior. He is talking about self-control, or better yet, our lack of submission to the will of God. All the examples cited are examples of those who do not typically practice self-control. It is this lack of self-control that Paul is addressing.

Those who refuse to see themselves on this list have taken their dedication to the truth only so far and then become comfortable with where they are. It is easy for any of us to deceive ourselves into believing that we are "mostly sin free." We do this in many ways, surrounding ourselves with people of like mind and also "like sin." We reinterpret or ignore scripture (and even the leading of the Holy Spirit) to make ourselves comfortable with a version of lesser truth. We set up judges for ourselves that are not listening to the Spirit of God, and don't have a clear understanding of the truth, nor are seeking the truth above all else.

Those cited on this list have another common condition, and that is one of self-obsession. Paul is telling us we are often self-obsessed. Paul is not trying to condemn us here, but to wake us up to the truth of who we are. Those on this list have demanded their own rights and close their eyes to their own shortcomings. Paul does not minimize sin, but rather makes sin an all-inclusive fact of the flesh. This is not the end of the thought. In fact, it is only the beginning.

He then helps us understand what he is saying by continuing with, "...And such were some of you (this list could have been expanded a little, and Paul may well of written, and such were ALL of you); but you were washed, but you were sanctified, but you were justified in the name of the Lord Jesus Christ, and in the Spirit of our God."

The "buts" here are very important. They connect our previous condition with our current one. Paul is saying that we WERE condemned, BUT now we are not because we have been washed, sanctified and justified. These are three separate experiences, and Paul isolated them each and lets them stand on their own.

"We have been washed clean of our sins."

"We have been sanctified by the sacrifice of Christ."

"We have been justified by God," who has placed on us the holy mantle of Christ. This is our current condition and it is one that is undeserved (washed), and it is unsought (sanctified), and it is unearned (justified).

We are unrighteous without the judgment of God to declare us so through Christ. Paul uses three descriptive terms for Jesus; the "Lord Jesus Christ." He is our Master (Lord), he is our brother (Jesus) and he is our Savior (Christ). As such, he is able to protect us, understand us, and save us from a selfish demise.

Then Paul brings this discussion into perspective by writing, "All things are lawful for me, but not all things are profitable."

Paul is once again, declaring his freedom in Christ not to be bound by the restrictions of sin. He is saying that he can do anything because he is no longer defined by his sinful condition. His relationship with Christ is what defines his standing before God. He is refusing to play the guilt game. Paul has a healthy perspective on what it means to be totally and utterly forgiven for his sins and his sinful condition. Yet with this knowledge he also understands something else of vast importance. He should also take advantage of the resources available to him to be out from under the control of sin. He continues, "All things are lawful for me, but I will not be mastered by anything."

Even though we are free from the legal reprisal of our actions. Even though we have come before a judge who is merciful and have an advocate who will declare us righteous, we still should seek not to be controlled by our lusts and desires. We should desire to be controlled by the spirit, not for legal reasons, nor to escape condemnation, but because it is expedient for us to do so. Just because we can, does not mean we should indulge. When our liberty distracts us from our relationship with God, then it is time to say, "Enough is enough!"

We can place ourselves under the control of God, not by combating sin, but by embracing Christ. Our focus should not be on ourselves and on our "rights" but rather on our relationship with Jesus. His leading is not inhibited by convention. His grace more than makes up for our shortfall.

Embrace the truth of Christ and do not let yourself be satisfied with lesser reflections or shadows. Admit your sinful nature and trust in your relationship with God through your Savior. God initiated it, and God is the one who will keep and sustain it. "For you have been bought with a price, and there are none who can snatch you from God's hand."

Transgender Living Without Sexual Reassignment Surgery (SRS)

Can I Create A Balance?

A Grace-filled Perspective of a Male to Female Transgender

Q: Can I create an emotional balance through cross-dressing?

Those who cross-dress due to gender identity typically try to present a believable image. For a male trying to look female, this usually involves padding (and padding some more), shaving (and then shaving again), plucking, pulling, tweezing, cinching, taping, and applying lots of carefully chosen make-up. Then comes the struggle into an outfit which emphasizes certain curves, and de-emphasizes others. The results can be very convincing, but they only last a few hours before the beard starts to appear, and the tape loosens. This presentation is temporary and the more permanent solution of surgery including sexual reassignment surgery (SRS) is one that only a few transgender people have the resources to pursue.

The idea of the magic pill that would just change how you look is commonly shared. Medical science now can create a fairly believable presentation, if the individual is willing to commit to the process.

How many surgeries might it take to change a male body into a permanent believable female form? What would it cost to re-sculpt a male into a female presentation achieved now through make-up and forms? Plenty!! All that fat in the midsection would have to be moved down to the butt and thighs. Electrolysis, breast implants, more electrolysis, eyelid-lifts, rib removal, voice box surgery, lip enhancement, face-lift, hair implants, diet, hormones, and years of counseling before and after. Even after all that, the hands would still be large, and so would the feet.

The term "SRS" makes it sound so neat and easy. However, the process takes years and hundreds of thousands of dollars to do the job properly. (For those who have dedicated themselves to this route, it is no easy journey!)

Most transgender will have to be content with the occasional cross-dressing experience. Since SRS is not a workable option where does that leave us? The non-op transgender person usually feels caught between two worlds. Not able to escape one gender, or really able to embrace the other.

Q: Do we really have to choose one gender over the other?

Even though we live in a largely polarized gender society, everyone has within them a male and female persona. The trans individual is acutely aware of this. Many in our mainstream communities, have declared a cross-dressing expression "wrong," or in Christian circles, "sinful." For the person born outwardly male but who inwardly feels female, expressing the feminine side in our western culture is difficult. These people learn to repress their female tendencies at an early age. By the time they are adults, their ignored female self has become twisted and scared like a child locked in a closet. A boy who tries to share in the female experience is ridiculed by his peers for the attempt: "Boys don't play with dolls!" "You throw like a girl!" "Don't be such a sissy!" "Boys don't cry!" Our society declares males to be strong and females to be weak. So the male who demonstrates female attributes is viewed as defective, weak or wrong.

Why do most people feel repelled by those who wish to change gender, even for a time? One reason this issue conjures up such intense emotion is because everyone's identity, or place in society, is determined by comparisons. We need to compare ourselves, one to another, in order to define who we are. (ie: male vs female - rich vs poor - etc.) When we cross-dress, we not only change the way the world views us, but how it views itself. As a result, the man who says it's "OK" to act like a woman rocks the societal boat in such a way that all of us in the boat start to lose our balance. Our western culture NEEDS to polarize the genders to keep woman and men in their places!

I do NOT believe that this view of gender is consistent with the teachings of

Christ. This view is especially harmful for those of us who feel that we are both male and female, or occupy a different niche on the gender spectrum.

For many transgender, the two voices inside are equally loud. Trying to give heed to both the female and male voice is difficult. Unfortunately, for the Christian, there is often a lethal and powerful third voice. It is the voice of self-condemnation. This voice gets its authority from a warped societal view of gender polarity and some Biblical scripture taken out of context. This voice I call, "the religious impostor."

This religious imposter has taken the concept of polarized gender in a dangerous direction. Not only is the desire to cross-dress viewed as wrong, but also as against God's law. In fact, this third voice believes that cross-dressing is so bad, if exposed or even mentioned, all it holds dear will be lost not only in this life now, but in the life to come. It is the role of this third voice to make sure the closet door stays closed. This "religious imposter" is arrogant, self-inflated, legalistic, depressed, confused, and above all else, scared.

The religious imposter is not without historical peers. He has been with us for thousands of years. He appears in every encounter throughout scripture between Jesus Christ and the Pharisees. What does Jesus have to say about this imposter? In Matthew 23, Jesus says, "You tie up heavy loads and lay them on men's shoulders . . . you shut off the kingdom of Heaven . . . for you do not enter in yourselves, nor do you allow those who are entering to go in. You blind guides . . . How often I wanted to gather you . . . the way a hen gathers her chicks under her wings, and you were unwilling."

We need to break free from this religious imposter. He is the one who would keep us from a loving relationship with our God. "God demonstrates His own love towards us, in that while we were yet sinners, Christ died for us!" (Romans: 5) Jesus calls us as we are. He desires nothing on our part other than acceptance of his grace and his righteousness. Is this hard to understand? Jesus wants us to come to him as little children. He wants to gather us up. No strings attached.

The female inside wishes for this with all of her heart. Because you have repressed her for so many years, she is still very much a child. She has no real history, no job and no bills to pay. She is truly free from any responsibility. Perhaps that is one of the reasons why it feels so good when you cross-dress? Your male-self, on the other hand, has a long history, but now feels frustrated and hollow. However, the good news is it does not have to be this way!

Its time to start to undo some of the damage caused by polarized gender.

FIRST. Don't be so hard on yourself. If you are like me, then you never meant to be legalistic or unloving. You truly thought that by fighting your transgender nature you were doing the right thing. Move past that! Accept who you are right now, and embrace the grace that God has freely given you.

> *"Come to me all who are weary and heavy-laden, and I will give you rest, . . . my yoke is easy and my burden is light." (Matthew: 11)*

SECOND. Let the little girl out to play. She really needs some clean fresh air. Do not try and justify it; just know that this is who you are inside and accept it. Take lots of deep breaths!!! She is still a child and has yet to experience the world. Your male self has already been down this path and can help her along, like a father helps guide a daughter.

THIRD. Realize it is the Lord's will for you to be whole. Jesus prayed on behalf of his followers for this very thing. One such prayer was "that we would all be one; even as the Father and Jesus are one." (John: 17) Jesus knows the importance of unity. He knows the importance of being honest with yourself. Jesus wants you to be a whole and honest child of God.

FOURTH. Reject your "religious imposter." Your relationship with God is what has saved you, but your imposter needs to somehow add to the work of the cross. Realize that you will never be "good enough" to earn God's favor, it is a FREE gift, and cannot be purchased by you. The religious imposter inside is a neurotic perfectionist that never feels he can be right with God. His compulsion to feel safe with God fuels an unhealthy desire for perfection. His endless compulsive, legalistic, and moralistic self-evaluation makes it impossible to feel accepted before God. His perception of personal failure leads to a loss of self-esteem and triggers anxiety, fear and depression. Call him to account. Don't be ruled by fear any longer.

FIFTH. Don't be afraid to discover your true self. Integrate your male and female selves whenever possible. Don't try and hide from either of them. As you are able, integrate. This can be done in little ways.

SIXTH. Resist the temptation to self-annihilate. Write a letter from your male self to your female self, and let her know what he likes about her.

Write a letter from your female self to your male self and let him know what she likes about him.

SEVENTH. Surrender control of your life and trust in God's grace. You have condemned yourself under the harsh rule of law. Realize, however, that the price was already paid by Jesus. Trust that God's purpose for you is not to be destroyed, but to experience fellowship and joy.

EIGHTH. Realize that this is a roller coaster ride. It will make you feel sick to your stomach if you try and fight the turns and twists. So try to relax and enjoy the ride for what it is.

May I suggest a book for you? It is *Abba's Child* by Brennan Manning (Navpress). The author puts forth a compelling argument for "grace living." Enjoy.

Weighing our Options

Thoughts about making purposeful choices.

Q: What Sort of Choices Do We Really Have?

Have any of you ever noticed that the flow of life often sweeps us in unexpected directions? You might answer, “Duh, this is not news. Why point out the obvious?”

I bring it up because we often continue in this flow without realizing we have other choices. We think we have made a determined choice when we choose between two or three options, even when what we want to do or desire is not on that list.

“So...what do you want for lunch dear?”

To this question the options presented might be, “You can have the tuna sandwich, or the ham.” We respond by making a choice limited to the options presented. Perhaps we chose the ham only because we hate tuna. Most of our life is spent choosing between options, none of which we ever desired for ourselves. When we choose the ham sandwich, we may think a profound personal choice has been made, but in reality we are only choosing between the limited options available.

What about faith? As with the ham and tuna, are we choosing only between the options available? Are we going with the flow or investigating for ourselves what the truth of who God really is? Are we pursuing an honest relationship with God, or just eating a tuna sandwich? When we investigate, are we merely trying to decipher between existing options and the points-of-view of others, or are we exploring original thought?

Consider the questions asked of Jesus in the New Testament. Those alive in Jesus' day rarely asked him a "completely authentic" question. As a result, most of his answers were confusing because the questions asked were not very relevant to the real issue at hand. He did not ignore the question, but looked through the question into the life and motives of the person asking it. Although the questions were often trivial, his answers were not. Jesus was able to find an authentic truth hidden within the question. He seldom chose tuna or ham.

A question asked of him once revolved around the query as to the suffering of a person born with a handicap, "Who was at fault, him, his father or his mother?" You will notice that Jesus did not answer that question directly but rather used the question to try and convey a worthwhile point about the nature of God. His answer was, "Neither. This person was born this way in order that God may be manifested in him."

This was a typical response for Jesus because so many (if not all) the questions asked of him were asked from a societal perspective that Jesus did not share. He was not being evasive, but was trying to redeem the question by illuminating a real worthwhile issue. I find it curious that we had God incarnate on Earth, and could not think up any worthwhile questions to ask!

We are not just Republicans or Democrats, but voters. I am not only male or female but also a person. The limited definitions of male and female offered in our culture are too restrictive for most. Rather than explore an original self definition of personhood, most people try to squeeze themselves into the polarized roles of male or female.

For those who identify as transgender, the incongruity between our socially perceived gender and our self-determined gender is the primary catalyst for Gender Identity Disorder (GID). When we embrace society's limited definition of gender (of what it means to be male and female) we severely limit our ability to learn or realize the truth of who we are. We choose between these limited options out of fear of social rejection; fear of losing our livelihoods; fear of risking stigma.

Even though most attempt to exist in our society by following its rules, an increasing number of individuals are rejecting their social conditioning. They see flaws in our western gender construct, but the ability to chart a different course is difficult because the only social compass we possess resists pointing in the right direction.

We are social creatures and early on in our lives (from birth really) we attempt to "fit in." Even though we are frustrated by our inability to fully fit in, the biggest frustration we feel does not come from this inability, but rather from the fact that we feel we have no workable alternatives. Where are the other choices? We have difficulty imagining choices beyond tuna or ham. Our fear keeps us from exploring options other than male and female, because we were not raised understanding those options.

There has been some minor progress made on developing a better concept of gender. Someday, hopefully society will evolve to a state that will unilaterally embrace a more open godly perspective about gender that includes acceptance and diversity. But for those who grew up in the 50s, 60s and 70s, we have difficulty embracing options beyond male and female. How can we be saved from this wretched state?

There is an answer. As always, it is found in the life and teachings of Jesus. He can help us pursue an honest personhood outside of our gender. Because Jesus loves and accepts us as we are, we can embrace who we are, and find our true selves in the pursuit of Him. A relationship with Christ changes us fundamentally. The freedom in Christ to explore ourselves and our world should be one that is unfettered.

The power of sin that Christ frees us from is more than just us choosing to limit or change some unwanted actions or thoughts. "Is it right or wrong?" "Is it sin or not?" Jesus has set us free from the power of those questions that attempt (in the asking) to supersede our self-determination. We can create or discover more options if we give up our fears and embrace unfettered grace. The real power of the cross is to defeat the agenda of sin in our life (which attempts to limit us) and replace it with a highly-valued personhood that can lead to an honest exploration of godly life-changing choices. We may never fully appreciate the depth of forgiveness, or the freedom and profound purpose found in grace.

In the T-community there is a lot of emphasis placed on "who we really are." Who we really are as people goes beyond our gender. Don't let limited available options hold you back. If we embrace grace for ourselves and we may discover who we "really are" in Christ.

When we play a game, we usually try to win. Life is no game, yet we mistakenly play it as if we trying NOT to lose. (For those who follow football, they know that the "prevent defense" often results in a disappointing loss.) Let go of the fear and explore your options, knowing that you are a child of God. As such, the victory is already yours.

This year make a choice that is honestly yours, make a godly choice.

Questions from a Conservative Pastor to a Christian Cross-dresser

These are actual questions sent to Light in the Closet from a pastor of a conservative mainstream denominational church. One of his questions reference what he identifies as "sin." Light in the Closet does not hold to the same view of sin as this pastor. However, it was necessary to reference sin in order to communicate in a way this minister would understand. His questions, although designed to be argumentative, deserve careful answers that communicate. LITC hopes that these responses will help our readers be prepared with solid arguments when being confronted.

Q: *How does your cross-dressing promote God's image and your acceptance of who God has made you (in relation to your gender)?*

There is no quick answer to that, nor one that applies to all situations. My answer would be different within different contexts depending on the age, faith and gender of the person asking the question.

The first part of your question, "How does cross-dressing promote God's image?"

I suppose it promotes it in terms of witness. Cross-dressing has allowed me access to a group of individuals that are largely shunned by the Church. This I consider a calling and a ministry. God put this calling on my heart ten years ago, and has yet to remove the burden and love I feel for the LGBTQI+ community. When I am dressed in a female persona, I try to portray a realistic image.

What I hope will come through is my humanity. I am not ignorant to the fact that the lines are a bit blurred, but I am trying to find my way (without much of a cultural road map, only the life of Christ) by relying on God's Spirit moment by moment. Hopefully, the image of God that comes through is one of acceptance and love. This is the image of God that I am trying to portray to a group of individuals who have experienced much rejection and condemnation. I hope the image I portray says to those in the LBGTQ+ community, that they are not outside of God's love because of their lifestyle or failings, nor outside of God's care. This image of God (loving, welcoming, forgiving) stands in stark contrast to the one being promoted by some of the mainstream churches that insist on pointing out the failings of others especially in areas where they themselves do not struggle. The image of God, (what it means to be like Jesus) which I promote has more to do with partnering with others, to say to them, "Hey world! I know that God loves me as I am, and He loves you too!"

The second part: "How does cross-dressing promote...your acceptance of who God has made you (in relation to your gender)?"

It may be hard to explain this part, since you have not had to deal with my life or my thorns. But let me give it a shot.

I'm laughing to myself (about myself) at this point because what God has led me to in regards to self-acceptance is something I could never have guessed going into this process. I was raised to think the only way to overcome a problem was to face it head on and do battle with it (onward Christian soldiers). If that did not work, then I would use the cut and run method of fleeing from a situation so I would not be tempted. The problem I found with both these methods is that my actions were based on MY EFFORT and that, as it turns out, limited or undercut the actions and work of God. I thought I knew what God wanted for me (based on scripture and teaching), but I did not know that my interpretations, and those of my church, were by default culturally motivated. (I speak about what defines a male and a female.) Our cultural definitions of male and female become intertwined with what we read in the Bible.

Our cultural filters interpret the scriptures in a way that is more palatable to our current day sensibilities, wants and desires. Reading scripture within our cultural context can often lead to a poor translation and therefore poor application of what it is that God intended.

Since I was raised in the Church my understanding of what it meant to be a male was garnered from both a social and a Biblical perspective. The cultural ideal of male was blended into my understanding of what God expected of me as a male. This created within my young mind a rather uncomfortable self-image where my natural desires towards the female role were viewed by me as wrong, evil or sinful. I equated my lack of understanding of the male mindset as a failing on my part. I began a life-long process of weeding out those female expressions and desires by trying to eliminate them. I learned early on to suppress my feelings and hide my thoughts (and even my actions). This I thought was the right thing to do.

I did not realize at the time that sometimes the only way through a valley is THROUGH the valley. I had no idea when I was battling these feelings that I was doing myself grave emotional harm. Although my intentions were to become "right with God," what I ended up doing was shutting down so much of myself that I lost who I was in the process. This I thought was perhaps what it meant to die to myself. I was VERY wrong.

Confessing our sins also means to acknowledge the reality of who we are. My acceptance of my female side has allowed me to accept myself and realize how much I need God. Accepting my female side, and the exploration of that, has allowed me to explore aspects of my humanity that I was afraid to express (creative, emotional, nurturing).

This process of rediscovery has helped heal some very deep and painful wounds. I laugh about this part because, interestingly enough, my acceptance of my female side has led to self-acceptance, and an understanding of my humanity and also the acceptance of my MALE side as well. I am enjoying more peace now between my male and female expressions than I had ever thought possible. Confessing my failings, my sins, and myself to God has led to a real death to self (a preconceived notion of who I thought I should be) and allowed me to take ownership of who I really am before God and what my role is as a child of God.

God is at work exposing and redeeming my sin nature, both male and female. My wounds are laid bare, and real healing can commence.

Q: *"Could you say that cross-dressing is a way to express your confusion about who you are and God's design for your life?"*

I think I answered some of this already. But to elaborate, let me also say that I had mistakenly viewed cross-dressing as a sin. I am very confident that I am living the life now that God has intended. I was confused about my gender, but that confusion was only a manifestation of a much deeper issue I needed to work on. God did have a plan for my life which involved me understanding my personhood. Cross-dressing helped me to clear up some of that confusion by allowing me to tap into a part of my personality that I was suppressing. In that respect it has been a therapeutic tool to gain understanding about God's intentions and design for me. Embracing my full gender draws me closer to the one who created me.

Q: *You use scripture to back up your experience. Could it be that your expressed transgender nature is a sin nature that needs to be re-coursed and restored in reference to God's primary intention for your life? God made male and female (different needs, expressions, body parts, etc.) - He never made man out of the context of these two genders.*

Let me correct your first statement when you say that I am "using" scripture to back up my experience. This is simply not true. I look to scripture for insights and to understand a biblical perspective. Most of my articles have come from insights or surprises that I have encountered while causally reading the bible. The application of those surprise scriptures comes well after the exploration. My take on Matthew 19 for example (page 43) was possible because after accepting my trans nature, my perspective or vision had widened making a new revelation accessible. I could simply say, "Hey, read the Bible, it's all in there."

You also asked, "Could it be?" Perhaps it could, for if you read my writings carefully, you will see that I never try to excuse my actions, nor do I say I am without faults in their expressions. I am very comfortable being imperfect. My goals are not crowns and accolades, but rather contributing heart-felt service to God and others. To stare honestly at all of yourself is not for the faint of heart. Ever heard the disclaimer, "Children do not try this at home. We are trained professionals?" I would have to echo that sentiment.

Although I have learned so much, most of it as through fire, I would not wish this path on anyone. In fact, I am trying to leave trail markers so that others will have an easier time of it.

Yes, it could be that my sin nature (I would say faults) needs to be re-coursed. I hope you feel the same way about your sin nature. Citing a particular bent that someone else has as more sinful than ours, only serves to justify our own failings. It clouds our ability to see our own faults clearly. I suppose that is the point though: To turn the spotlight off yourself and on to another? Jesus called this obsessing over the splinter in their eye while ignoring the log in our own.

The good news is that redemption has already taken place. We live in grace, and that has freed us to do meaningful loving things for others without fear of a misstep. For I have learned, through much pain, that ALL I do falls short of the mark (what sin actually is) and I am okay with that. I allow the spirit inside me to mature the fruits of the spirit so I may enjoy those fruits when they ripen.

We may disagree on this issue due to our personal experiences. We may also need to navigate word semantics and a basic Biblical understanding to have a healthier discourse. It may be a bridge too far, but I hope your prayers are for God's design to be revealed.

Do not confuse my self-acceptance with total self-approval. I am not deluded as to the reality of my faults, and I accept the responsibility for my actions. I know I am an imperfect person saved by grace. I also know, however, that there are people out there struggling with issues that are not easily resolved, living under a burden that has suppressed and twisted them into a state of inactivity. We are to live the abundant life, and these people have been placed under a false weight that only serves to crush them. Jesus died to set us free from the power of sin, to never again become a slave to the agenda of sin. I would love to hear that preached from the pulpit.

I also know that those who think themselves righteous are righteous only through comparisons with others they perceive to be weaker than themselves. It's not unlike the pretty girl who surrounds herself with ugly friends. She feels that she looks good in contrast, but is she really prettier (more righteous) than those she compares herself to?

Your last point about male and female is more of a biological question than a Biblical one. Biologically there is a wonderful range of body types that manifest in the size, height and build of each person in a completely unique way. Gender is very similar in that although categorized in the Western world as mainly male and female, the types of gender expression vary widely. Without getting too graphic, many are born with ambiguous genitalia and although these are labeled either male or female in our culture, most other cultures allow for a healthy recognition of a third gender.

As you know, the roles of men and women are culturally driven. God has cited roles for male, female, and saris, as well as rich, poor, slave and free. Some of these are applicable today, others were descriptions of social conditions at the time. God works with what we offer trying to communicate with us in ways we can understand.

God is very patient in this. I hope we followers show each other the same patience and understanding when it comes to communication and give each other the benefit of the doubt.

What is the Nature of God's Heart?

Jesus Talks about Acceptance, Love and Grace

(A look at Luke 15-17)

Light in the Closet strongly believes that God works in a unique way with each child of God. We sometimes have very little tolerance for those whose differences make us uncomfortable. All of God's children have value and dignity, and it is wrong for any of us to deny dignity to our brothers and sisters. It is dangerous to judge someone else because the motives behind the actions are hard to see. Some, like the Biblical prodigal son in Luke chapter 15, take advantage of their relationship with God, squandering what God bestows on them. The prodigal son was driven by his passions and lusts, yet God ran to meet him and welcomed him home even though he was only returning to satisfy his physical hunger.

The Prodigal Son - Amazing Love, Amazing Grace

The story of the prodigal son was told by Jesus in response to complaints by the scribes and Pharisees. The Pharisees were upset with Jesus because he associated with tax gatherers and sinners. I am convinced that many who say they follow Christ today, if they heard Jesus preach and saw who he associated with, would have serious objections as well.

In Luke 15 we read:

> *"Now all the tax collectors and the sinners were coming near Him to listen to Him. Both the Pharisees and the scribes began to grumble, saying, "This man receives sinners and eats with them."*

It is a fact that Jesus went into places that were "off limits" to the respectable people of that day. He ate in the homes of people of low reputation and with those whom everyone agreed were sinners. Some today try to quantify this behavior by claiming that each of these encounters resulted in everyone present turning from their sinful ways and that Jesus knew this ahead of time so therefore these people really were more like unripe fruit that Jesus was picking. Sorry, that does not really cut it. Those who knew Jesus then and watched his ministry knew better. The Pharisees did not accuse Jesus of associating with sinners, because these people became "good tithe-paying Jews."

What was Jesus's attitude towards those who were sinners? This becomes evident as we continue in Luke 15:

> *"So He told them this parable, saying, 'What man among you, if he has a hundred sheep and has lost one of them, does not leave the ninety-nine in the open pasture and go after the one which is lost until he finds it? When he has found it, he lays it on his shoulders, rejoicing. And when he comes home, he calls together his friends and his neighbors, saying to them, 'Rejoice with me, for I have found my sheep which was lost!' "I tell you that in the same way, there will be more joy in heaven over one sinner who repents than over ninety-nine righteous persons who need no repentance."*

Wow Jesus! Shouldn't I also be rejoiced over? Since I am not lost that would make me one of those righteous ninety-nine. Are you saying that the angels consider the one person who is lost more valuable than me and my ninety-eight friends. That does not seem fair to me. Please Jesus can you explain this more?

So Jesus does. Continuing in Luke 15 we read:

> *"Or what woman, if she has ten silver coins and loses one coin, does not light a lamp and sweep the house and search carefully until she finds it? When she has found it, she calls together her friends and neighbors, saying, 'Rejoice with me, for I have found the coin which I had lost!' In the same*

> *way, I tell you, there is joy in the presence of the angels of God over one sinner who repents."*

I don't know Jesus, that seems a bit vague. All of those ten coins had equal worth. Why would the one coin that was lost be more precious than the other nine? All those coins looked the same, they were identical and had equal value. Why does this woman make such an effort to find just one?

Jesus continues with one of his best-known stories, the prodigal son. In Luke 15 we read:

> *"And He said, "A man had two sons. The younger of them said to his father, 'Father, give me the share of the estate that falls to me ' So he divided his wealth between them. And not many days later, the younger son gathered everything together and went on a journey into a distant country, and there he squandered his estate with loose living. Now when he had spent everything, a severe famine occurred in that country, and he began to be impoverished. So he went and hired himself out to one of the citizens of that country, and he sent him into his fields to feed swine. And he would have gladly filled his stomach with the pods that the swine were eating, and no one was giving anything to him."*
>
> *But when he came to his senses, he said, 'How many of my father's hired men have more than enough bread, but I am dying here with hunger! I will get up and go to my father, and will say to him, "Father, I have sinned against heaven, and in your sight; I am no longer worthy to be called your son; make me as one of your hired men.' So he got up and came to his father. But while he was still a long way off, his father saw him and felt compassion for him, and ran and embraced him and kissed him. And the son said to him, 'Father, I have sinned against heaven and in your sight; I am no longer worthy to be called your son.'*
>
> *But the father said to his slaves, 'Quickly bring out the best robe and put it on him, and put a ring on his hand and sandals on his feet; and bring the fattened calf, kill it, and let us eat and celebrate; for this son of mine was dead and has come to life again; he was lost and has been found.' And they began to celebrate.*
>
> *Now his older son was in the field, and when he came and*

approached the house, he heard music and dancing. And he summoned one of the servants and began inquiring what these things could be. And he said to him, 'Your brother has come, and your father has killed the fattened calf because he has received him back safe and sound.'

But he became angry and was not willing to go in; and his father came out and began pleading with him. But he answered and said to his father, 'Look! For so many years I have been serving you and I have never neglected a command of yours; and yet you have never given me a young goat, so that I might celebrate with my friends; but when this son of yours came, who has devoured your wealth with prostitutes, you killed the fattened calf for him.'

And he said to him, 'Son, you have always been with me, and all that is mine is yours. But we had to celebrate and rejoice, for this brother of yours was dead and has begun to live, and was lost and has been found.'"

This story has been visited and revisited thousands of times by many preachers. Some call this the watermark of perfect repentance. They claim that the prodigal son left the depravity of the world (the pig sty) pulled himself up and made the long journey back home, contrite and fully aware of the magnitude of his sin. The son was repentant and deeply sorry for his actions and came to his father expecting nothing but scorn and a place with the servants. Wow what a humble spirit! But, the father in his mercy ran to greet him and gave him a reward for his effort of contrition and the long road back he traveled to get right with him. Gee, how neatly this fits into the legalistic mentality. I understand why it is often interpreted this way, but those who push this interpretation I believe are dead wrong! That interpretation is out of context, and way off the mark.

Let's look at the "whole" teaching of Jesus. What was his intent? What do the other two stories have to do with the prodigal son story? Are these random stories that Jesus was telling? Or, was Jesus using these three stories to answer the accusations of the Pharisees and teach relevant truth? I go with the latter.

So what was Jesus addressing? We see that tax gathers were coming to Jesus to listen to what he had to say. (The lowest of the low to the Jewish people of that day. These were Jewish turn-coats who worked for the Roman government, excised large taxes from their friends and family, and kept huge amounts for themselves. The closest thing we have in today's society would be criminals who demand paid protection from store owners. Also, the "sinners" were coming to him (pretty much everyone else). This distinction is very telling. Why not just state that Jesus was befriending sinners? Wouldn't that cover everyone anyway? Why the distinction?

It is clear from this statement that the Jews believed in a hierarchy of sin. The tax gatherers were considered the lowest of the low, beyond redemption and association. It was difficult for them to see Jesus in the company of sinners in general (prostitutes, deviants, and low-life) but to be with a tax-gatherer! Why did the tax gatherers occupy the lowest rung? Because they effected the Pharisees and scribes in the most direct way. They went toe-to-toe with them, disrespected them and demanded vast amounts of money and goods. The tax gatherers stole from the Jewish people which affected their ability to tithe. They usurped the authority of the Pharisees. To most of the Jewish people, these tax-gatherers were beyond redemption and wholly outside the Jewish communities.

Through these three stories, Jesus addresses the issue of acceptance of sinners in general and the incorrect idea that some in society had less worth than others.

All in God's Family are Precious

Jesus starts by telling the story of the lost sheep. All the sheep belong to the same flock and are therefore members of the same family. They belong to a community that travels together and is under the watchful eye of the shepherd. In this story, one sheep out of one hundred is lost. The shepherd looks diligently until he finds that sheep, grabs it, flings it across his shoulders and carries it all the way back to the flock. Jesus is saying to his accusers, Look, we are all part of the same family. If one of our family members is lost, I am going to do what it takes to bring them back, even if I have to carry him all the way myself!

OK, great lesson Jesus. I get it, we are all Jews and we should all be together. I may not agree, but I get it.

All Have Equal Value and Worth

Then Jesus turns it up a notch. He tells another story about ten coins. The first story had one hundred sheep, and there was only one ba-a-a-d one among them. Now in this story a woman has only ten coins, ALL of equal value. Why the drop in amounts? It is harder to ignore one in ten as it would be one in one hundred. In the story, the woman drops a coin, and cleans the whole house until she finds it.

As in the first story, there is much rejoicing over the one that was found. We may have questioned the value of the one sheep lost, but all of these coins have equal value. Jesus is saying that all of us (no matter how awful our sins) have the exact same value. This addresses the idea that some sins or sinners are worse than others. Jesus is saying that we are all the same and no one is outside of redemption.

Wow Jesus, that is pretty radical. When is lunch being served? Got any fish and bread handy? We would like to see you do that food miracle again!

God's Love is Radical

Jesus is not finished though. Next he tells the story of the prodigal son. Although he is the youngest son, he has the audacity to ask his father for his inheritance early. This is curious on a couple of levels. He was the "younger" son and the bulk would have normally fallen to the older son. However, the father divides the inheritance equally between the two boys, which is not the norm culturally. The Jewish people of the day would have seen this as a terrible breach in etiquette. And the message of Jesus that all those in the family deserve the same inheritance would be unmistakable. Normally in Jewish culture, the eldest daughter would have to be married before the younger, and the older son would have gotten his inheritance before the younger (if the younger received any at all). In this story, this very kind father agrees to the son's request and gives him the full share.

What does this son do with his wealth? He squanders it on loose living and whores. Imagine if you will, listening to Jesus back then and hearing these words come out of his mouth. This disrespectful son is not much of a son at all. He is driven by his lusts, greed and a willingness to reject all the good advice his father has to offer. Yet the father gives him an inheritance anyway.

I've often heard people say, "If grace is so powerful and people can be forgiven for anything they do, then what keeps people from sinning? You have to repent first and not sin anymore to be saved. If grace were totally free, then we would want to continue to do those things we enjoy and are tempted by. There has to be accountability!"

Jesus's answers to these questions are filled with radical grace. In the story of the prodigal son, there is very little accountability. There is, however, dire consequences for this young man's choices.

In the story, the son eventually runs out of money and is forced to find work. Having no skills to speak of, he ends up doing the worst job imaginable, and though he apparently tries to be self-sufficient is not able to make enough of an income to even feed himself.

At this point, the boy becomes hungry and his stomach begins to growl. He remembers the graciousness of his father and how much better his father treated his workers than his boss was treating him. Even though he was probably embarrassed to go, his appetite is strong, and he comes up with a plan. "I will tell my father that I know because of my actions that I do not deserve to be his son anymore. Maybe I could ask him to give for a job. Hey, who knows, that might work!"

On a personal note, I have to question his motives. His appetites drove him away from his father, and apparently his appetite has turned his attention towards home. I don't see this trek towards home as a perfect picture of repentance. It was his desire to be fed that put him on the road home. He recognized that his father could meet his need, and even though his motives were selfish, the fact that he turned to his father for help was enough for his father to respond.

The story goes on. "While the son was still a long way off, his father saw him and felt compassion for him, and ran and embraced him and kissed him." The father was anxiously awaiting his son's return. I picture the father in the highest tower of his home continually gazing towards the horizon for any sign of the child. How long was the son gone? How long did the father sit there waiting? Would it not have been prudent for the father, if he was so interested, to have one of his servants take on the task of lookout? No, it is the father himself that sits and eagerly waits. As soon as he catches a glimpse of the son on the road, "while he was still a long way off" the father runs out of the house and races towards him, hugs him, and kisses him.

The son then goes into his rehearsed speech intending to get yet something else from his father and says, 'Father, I have sinned against heaven and in your sight; I am no longer worthy to be called your son.' He intends to go on with the rest of the speech about becoming a hired hand and may have inquired as to when lunch might be served. But he is not able to finish the practiced speech. The father interrupts him and commands the servants there to quickly get the very best robe, new sandals, some bling (the ring was a sign of son-ship) and kill the fatted calf they had been preparing (perhaps for the son's hopeful return) and celebrate!

I've often wondered how effective this parenting style would be. I know with my children I tend to try and steer them towards positive choices. If one of my children behaved like the prodigal son, squandered what was his and then returned for more, I doubt that my response would be "welcome home!" I love my children but there are certain actions I would not put up with and those would have dire consequences if my children were to engage in them. My response to the return of the prodigal son might read more like this:

> *So the son returned to the father's home, came up to the door and knocked. The father had heard a rumor from a friend at work that day, that his delinquent son may be returning home. The knock at the door sent the father's heart racing at the thought that this might actually be him. He told a servant to answer the door and the servant came back a bit nervous and said, "Master, your son has returned."*
>
> *The father was surprised and wanted time to consider his response. He told the servant to have the son wait in his office for him. He told another servant to find the eldest brother who was out in the field working, so that they might discuss together what to do. The servant did what he was told.*
>
> *The older brother finally made it home, and the father and him considered together which course of action to take. Meanwhile, the prodigal son waited anxiously in the father's office while his stomach growled.*
>
> *Finally the father and the older brother enter the study. They are offended by the smell of this young man, who has been sleeping with pigs for the past few months. The father reels back, and gets angry at the servant for letting this boy into his office in such a condition. "Quick, take him outside and hose him off," the father demands, "Find one of his brother's old tunics to wear. And somebody, open a window!*
>
> *After the son is cleaned up enough to be let back in the house, the father finally grants him audience and listens to the full speech: "Father, I have sinned against heaven, and in your sight; I am no longer worthy to be called your son; make me as one of your hired men."*
>
> *"Is that it?" quips the Father. The father considers his son's proposal.*

The story would continue from there with some bartering and perhaps at some point the boy may get a meal. I doubt it would have been a free lunch. The boy would have to prove he was contrite and I'm sure a curfew, as well as other restrictions, would be part of their new arrangement. Most would agree that my version is better parenting, and a much more normal response.

This story is more about the character of God, than that of the son. Jesus uses this story to contrast the difference between us and God. God is much more loving, and forgiving than our sense of "fairness" would allow for. Jesus continues "his version" of the story with the elder brother's response.

Unlike my version, Jesus tells of an elder brother that discovers his younger delinquent brother is home only after the party has started. It is the sound of feasting that is his first clue. A feast he was not even invited to! He is very angry and confronts the father with the words, "this son of yours..." The father replies with the words, "He is your brother! Rejoice, he is home!"

In Jesus' version God is the father who is looking for any sign that we may turn to him. When he sees the smallest gesture on our part, the smallest inroad, the father comes running to meet us and ushers us into his home, gives us a gold ring, the finest clothing (the righteousness of God) to cover our stinky dirty frame, and throws the party to end all parties!

How deep is our Fathers love is for us! How much he desires for us to be with him. Is this good parenting? Perhaps not, but it is the heart of God and illustrates how ALL of God's children are equal and precious. It is God who looks for us. It is God who runs to us. It is God who carries us home.

I would love to stop the story here. It is a good ending. God loves us no matter what! However, there was another point Jesus addressed as well concerning the tax collectors.

Jesus Affirms the Value of the Tax Collector

In the Jewish culture, if someone in the family chose to go outside of the faith, or took up inappropriate activities or a lifestyle, the family would often disown him and could even go so far as have a funeral service for them. They were seen as having nothing to contribute and were totally shunned from the community. Jesus saw an opportunity to address this issue as well in the story of The Unrighteous Steward. In Luke 15 we read:

> *"Now He was also saying to the disciples, "There was a rich man who had a manager, and this manager was reported to him as squandering his possessions. And he called him*

and said to him, 'What is this I hear about you? Give an accounting of your management, for you can no longer be manager.'"

"The manager said to himself, 'What shall I do, since my master is taking the management away from me? I am not strong enough to dig; I am ashamed to beg. I know what I shall do, so that when I am removed from the management people will welcome me into their homes. And (so) he summoned each one of his master's debtors, and he began saying to the first, 'How much do you owe my master?'

And he said, 'A hundred measures of oil.' And he said to him, 'Take your bill, and sit down quickly and write fifty.' Then he said to another, 'And how much do you owe?' And he said, 'A hundred measures of wheat.' He said to him, 'Take your bill, and write eighty.'

And his master praised the unrighteous manager because he had acted shrewdly; for the sons of this age are more shrewd in relation to their own kind than the sons of light.

And I say to you, make friends for yourselves by means of the wealth of unrighteousness, so that when it fails, they will receive you into the eternal dwellings.

He who is faithful in a very little thing is faithful also in much; and he who is unrighteous in a very little thing is unrighteous also in much.

Therefore, if you have not been faithful in the use of unrighteous wealth, who will entrust the true riches to you? And if you have not been faithful in the use of that which is another's, who will give you that which is your own? No servant can serve two masters; for either he will hate the one and love the other, or else he will be devoted to one and despise the other. You cannot serve God and wealth."

Now the Pharisees, who were lovers of money, were listening to all these things and were scoffing at Him. And He said to them, "You are those who justify yourselves in the sight of men, but God knows your hearts; for that which is highly esteemed among men is detestable in the sight of God. The Law and the Prophets were proclaimed until

> *John; since that time the gospel of the kingdom of God has been preached, and everyone is forcing his way into it. But it is easier for heaven and earth to pass away than for one stroke of a letter of the Law to fail.*

I have recapped most all of the chapter because it really needs to be looked at in its entirety. In fact, the discourse continues with a reference to the divorce conversation he had earlier, and the importance of stewardship explored in the story of the rich man and the poor man.

But I will not go into those here. Instead, let us unpack this very curious story that at first doesn't seem to relate at all to the prodigal son.

The first three stories talked about all God's children having equal access, worth and value. No lifestyle or sin was outside of God's love and grace. Jesus also teaches us that there is no hierarchy of sin. Now Jesus goes into a story that has implications as to the motives behind the shunning of the tax gatherers. We read earlier that one of the main complaints of the Pharisees is that the tax gatherers were stealing funds from their treasuries. Jesus starts with this.

The parable of The Unrighteous Steward parallels what the tax gatherers were doing; collecting money, over charging, and keeping some for themselves. Basically they were stealing from the Romans and the Jewish people. They were living off of what was not rightfully theirs. Jesus tells of a dishonest manager who gets caught with his hand in the cookie jar. His master finds out about this and decides to fire him. Afraid for his welfare, this manager comes up with a plan to go to his master's debtors and get them to alter their bills to reflect less than they owe. He does this to get on their good side and is basically buying their friendship. The master finds out and although the manager is still fired, is impressed by the cleverness of the man.

At first glance, this story appears out of nowhere. Jesus through the story is saying, "Hey Pharisees, you can learn something about business from these tax gatherers. Yes, they are unrighteous, but they still have something to contribute." Jesus says it like this:

> *"...And his master praised the unrighteous manager because he had acted shrewdly; for the sons of this age are more shrewd in relation to their own kind than the sons of light. And I say to you, make friends for yourselves by means of the wealth of unrighteousness, so that when it fails, they will receive you into the eternal dwellings.*

Jesus is saying, yes I know they are sinners, but they still have something to offer. They are shrewd business people and you could learn a thing or two from them. These unrighteous people are stealing from each other, but at least are using their money to buy friendships and create associations. THAT IS BETTER THAN YOU ARE DOING! Wow Jesus, could you be harsher? Are you saying we should be like the tax gatherers? No, but Jesus is saying that they have value, if only to show us by contrast the true nature of our motives.

Jesus Also Cares for the Pharisees

Jesus then pointedly addresses the motive of the Pharisees and scribes:

> *"He who is faithful in a very little thing is faithful also in much; and he who is unrighteous in a very little thing is unrighteous also in much. Therefore, if you have not been faithful in the use of unrighteous wealth, who will entrust the true riches to you? And if you have not been faithful in the use of that which is another's, who will give you that which is your own?"*

Jesus, out of concern for the Pharisees, challenges them. He says they have been mishandling the money they have been entrusted with. If they cannot be trusted to handle material goods (that are God's tithes not theirs) then how can they be trusted to handle the important treasure like the priesthood of the people, and the spiritual well-being of the Jewish nation? He does not say this to anger them, but to challenge them to righteous accountability.

A few years later, Paul will write to the Roman church saying, "Therefore let us not judge one another anymore, but rather determine this -- not to put an obstacle or a stumbling block in a brother's way....Therefore you have no excuse, everyone of you who passes judgment, for in that which you judge another, you condemn yourself; for you who judge practice the same things.

Jesus is letting the Pharisees know that they are no better than, and in some ways worse than the tax collectors.

He goes on to say:

> *"No servant can serve two masters; for either he will hate the one and love the other, or else he will be devoted to one and despise the other. You cannot serve God and wealth."*

Again he has addressed their motives. Who do they serve? Why do they judge others? Is it because they want financial gain, or are they genuinely concerned with these lost souls? If the latter, why are the sinners being shunned? Why are the Pharisees not doing the work of God and opening a door to these fellow Jews?

The scripture finishes with:

> *"Now the Pharisees, who were lovers of money, were listening to all these things and were scoffing at Him. And He said to them, "You are those who justify yourselves in the sight of men, but God knows your hearts; for that which is highly esteemed among men is detestable in the sight of God.*
>
> *The Law and the Prophets were proclaimed until John; since that time the gospel of the kingdom of God has been preached, and everyone is forcing his way into it. But it is easier for heaven and earth to pass away than for one stroke of a letter of the Law to fail."*

Jesus affirms the law, but questions the motives of the Pharisees. He goes past the lesson of who is a sinner, and makes a straight-forward observation. Your motives are for personal gain, wealth and to gain social standing through self-righteous efforts. You may fool the community, but God knows your heart. Don't think you can force your way into Heaven.

Jesus loves us all. He loves those who think themselves righteous and those who know they are unrighteous. Jesus came into this world not to condemn the world, but so it may be saved through him.

> *"If anyone hears My sayings and does not keep them, I do not judge him; for I did not come to judge the world, but to save the world."*

Thoughts from a Male to Female Transgender/Cross-dresser

The following articles are written from the perspective of a cross-dresser (male to female). The experiences, feelings and insights expressed here are common to most cross-dressers. They may help in communicating your own feelings to your significant other, spouse, wife, children or other family members.

A Typical Story of a Male to Female Cross-dresser

For as far back as I can remember, I have wanted to be a girl. Early on I learned that this was not acceptable and so for most of my life I've struggled with this in secret. I grew up dreaming that if I wished hard enough when I went to sleep, I could awake as a girl.

When my parents realized my desire to express the feminine they disapproved. Their disapproval only helped to reinforce the need for secrecy it did not have any sway over my needs.

For the most part I think I was happy. I grew up doing typical male things but never really fit in. As I grew, I played sports and did the things most boys did, but it always felt like a struggle. Every chance I got, I would sneak into my sister's or mom's bedroom and try on some of their clothing.

I met my wife in high school, and thought that getting married would solve most of my issues. After a short stint in the army, I dove into a career had children and am now looking forward to grandchildren. I've been able to keep my desires for the most part hidden and separate from my "normal" life.

I really thought that as I got older my feelings would get easier to manage. Now that I am into mid-life, I have found just the opposite to be true. My desire to be and act feminine is greater than ever.

A couple of times I have dressed up to the nines for Halloween and other party events, and I often think about these times. I really wish I could do more, but I am afraid of the repercussions.

I love my wife and my children, but sometimes I feel like I will go crazy. I have not spoken to my wife or really anybody in an open and honest way regarding my true feelings about myself, because I know that they would disapprove.

So, I continue to do those things expected of me, but I am not sure how much longer I can keep this secret to myself.

If this sounds like you, then you are not alone!

There are many factors that go into the feelings we get when we cross-dress. A freedom through this self expression is a big one. Giving ourselves permission to express the mannerisms and emotions we normally attach to the "other" gender role is another. Escape from the daily commitments our male selves deal with is also huge.

When we are frustrated over something as basic as our gender, everything in our life will suffer. This dissatisfaction will almost certainly have you looking for comfort elsewhere. This usually means an increased desire to cross-dress and participate in those activities.

Most transgender experience a dramatic increase in their desire to cross-dress between the ages of 45-65. For most if not all, the idea of sexual reassignment surgery (SRS) seems an unavoidable eventuality, but not a workable reality. The fact is, this is the time when andropause begins (the male version of menopause). During andropause your hormones are changing radically. It is not unlike puberty.

It is important to find a therapist you can trust. Talking with a medical doctor is also a good idea. Remember, you are not alone in this.

Be warned though, many doctors will want to prescribe drugs or hormones right away. Doctors love drugs. If you think a pill has a chance of doing it for you, then they are more than willing to oblige. This, however, may not be the best course of action. Talk to a therapist first and make sure you know what all your options are. Your feelings, although very intense, may change after awhile and you should give them time to run their course. Take the time to weigh all your alternatives before making a radical life change.

Try to establish a personhood that makes sense to you and the gender expression that resonates best for you should follow. Discovering what your niche is along the gender spectrum is what will foster true self-acceptance and peace. What that eventually leads to needs to be unwrapped thoughtfully and carefully.

Try to accept yourself as you are now, and you will be able to make a better choice for the future. "Accepting yourself" can mean a lot of things. What does that mean to you?

Who Am I? A Search in the Mirror.

For a long time, I would look in the mirror and not recognize that the person I saw was me. I'm referring to that man with the beard. At times, I would actually be startled at the reflection in the mirror in much the same way as if a stranger had unexpectedly walked into the room.

It bothered me that I could not make friends with my reflection. Something was missing.

One day I purchased a wig, shaved and tried on some makeup. It was amazing to me how different I looked. Suddenly, I saw someone I could relate to staring back at me. The hair and the make-up were not real "glam" but more honest and natural. The reflection in the mirror looked like how I felt inside.

This was amazing to me. How could this image evoke such a strong emotional response?

I have since taken steps to incorporate that vision of my inner self into my everyday outward self. Slowly my male persona is looking more like the female I am inside. The beard is gone of course. Now I am working on skin care, wearing some makeup (well blended), gender-neutral looking clothes, coloring my hair, and plucking my eyebrows. The comments I get are mostly positive and that I look younger.

I am attempting to "own" my outward image. My "look" has changed, and my "outlook" has also. This has been great therapy.

Open Letters from a Cross-dresser

Following are three journal entries from a married man about his cross-dressing. He is a Christian, and what he shares may or may not resonate with the reader. LITC has left these offerings "as is" so the reader would get unedited insight into his unique experiences. (3 Journal Entries)

Entry 1: Struggling Alone

At first glance, I am very passable as a man (laugh). Am I a transsexual, or something else? I don't know. However I often wished I were a woman. No, I am not gay. In fact, I am fairly happy with my marriage.

I have been involved in Christian service most my life and a cross-dresser (cder) all my life. Although I've kept cding a secret, I didn't really see it as "sin" until I was in my teens. Unfortunately, I have spent decades fighting the impulse. I would plead before God to take away my feelings, and sometimes would earn some temporary relief from my desires. However, eventually I come back to the same point I start from. This is very confusing and very depressing. My pillow is often wet from my tears. My attitude of self-condemnation is equally matched by my self-loathing.

I've attempted to seek counseling for it but do not know where to go.

I always give time, money and talents to the Church and have witnessed boldly for our Lord. For the most part, it is just this one thing (cding) that I deal with. Aside from that, I appear to be the model Christian man.

I've successfully stuffed my feelings and desires a couple of times. I hoped this would please God. Unfortunately, I can only control my urges and desires at a great personal and spiritual cost. It involves shutting down not just those undesirable feelings, but most of my other emotions as well.

As a result, I've became rather despondent. I had to shut down so much of my God-given nature in order to control my feelings and urges, that not much is left now. Not only am I miserable, but I am making everyone around me miserable as well.

I still function during the week. I still try and do all the right things, but more and more I am feeling sick. The weekends are spent mostly in bed sleeping or watching TV. I'm very depressed, and my wife keeps pleading with me to get help.

I wish I could tell her what is really going on.

Entry 2: When I finally told her:

I'd been in a major funk for awhile. My wife kept hounding and hounding me trying to get me to open up. So one day through tears, I finally told her what was going on. She looked surprised, but stayed very calm. We talked late into the night.

The next day she called a counselor (for herself) who told her it wasn't her fault and that I may just be wired that way. I thought this would upset her, but it actually made it easier for her to talk to someone who was aware of transgender issues.

She has been extremely supportive, and has even let me explore my feminine side at home. I know how much of an effort this has been for her. I had tried to tell her a couple of times before by bringing up the subject, but she usually seemed to be turned off by it. I just felt like she would not understand or be receptive. I thought that perhaps she would even leave me. But I suppose it is different now that this is "my issue" and not some faceless stranger's struggle.

Her willingness to talk to me about it is such a relief. I know it still troubled her, but she loves me and is willing to work this out. I am very blessed to have someone who is so patient.

Entry 3: Looking back, looking forward:

I had fought so hard and so long to deny myself. Now that I have given up, it really doesn't matter if it is sin anymore. I am too tired to care. Isn't 40 years of pleading for deliverance enough? If God was not answering my prayers, then perhaps I was praying for the wrong thing.

I know that God is still in my life and will not let go.

I finally confessed to God that I tried to change, but was not able to be the man-of-God I think I was supposed to be. I was surprised when God answered back, "I never asked you to change. That was your idea not mine."

God has made me this way for a reason. I am not broken, but am starting to understand that God needs me as I am. Now that I can deal openly (at least somewhat) with my gender identity issue, I feel like a large weight has been lifted. Almost like being born again. God has freed me in much the same way as He freed the Apostle Paul from the worry about his thorn in the flesh (2 Corinthians 12).

Is it sin? Some would say "no." Some would say "yes." I'm not sure, but it does not feel like sin anymore. I just know that I am saved by grace regardless. I have a peaceful and thankful heart for my God's tender mercy.

If I could have changed it I would have. But I see my transgender orientation now as a gift of grace for which I am thankful.

Should I Tell?

When a person cross-dresses due to gender identity, there is a fundamental shift in their persona. Not only do they look radically different, but they are also perceived as a different person. This is very unsettling for those close to them and often difficult to accept.

We get our "sense of self" largely from those around us. We rely on the input of others for our identity: How they treat us, how they define us, and if we are accepted or not. We compare and contrast ourselves to others as well; how do they act compared to us, what level of education do they have compared to us, how does their career compare to ours, and especially what they look like compared to us. They, in turn, get their "sense of self" through input, comparisons and contrasts with us.

Someone who changes (even for a time) something as basic as their gender, changes not only how they are perceived, but also how others perceive themselves. A strong negative reaction to your cross-dressing by family, friends and co-workers has a lot to do with how the cross-dressing directly affects their identity.

If your cross-dressing is more than just a passing phase or secret sexual expression, and rooted instead in gender identity, then you may want to consider finding a way to give those around you a heads up.

Unfortunately, most disclosure happens through accidental discovery, and since there is usually no frame of reference to understand this unexpected information, the resulting reaction is usually negative. Most people think sexual affair, Jerry Springer, or worse. Although negative first impressions can be repaired, it is best to have a positive first impression. A thoughtful approach to disclosure, framed within a context that is understandable, has the potential of working out well. Please see the articles below about telling a spouse and children. The question you should ask yourself is, "Why do I want to tell?"

The when, where and why of telling someone about your gender identity issue.

Telling can be one of the scariest ideas a closeted cross-dresser ever entertains. It goes against their very fiber and conditioning. For older cross-dressers (cders) they have trained themselves NOT to tell, so the idea of divulging anything is even more frightening.

There is a certain amount of control in having a secret. When you cross-dress in secret, you feel as though you have ultimate control over something very personal. No one else has input into what you are doing and therefore no control over you in this area. This has a very real appeal for those who feel as though they have no control over their life. If someone feels they are a "victim of their life," then cross-dressing can be an escape from those limitations. You could be saying to yourself, "I may have no control over my situation, but I can always cross-dress." If you tell someone, then that total control is lost.

However, cross-dressing can be addictive, and so therefore how much self-control do you really have? Are you controlling the when, where and the degree of your cross-dressing, or is this compulsion controlling you? Although no one has control over you in this regard, do you really have ultimate control yourself? If your thoughts constantly turn to cross-dressing to the detriment of your other relationships, then you have a serious issue with either your gender identity, or out-of-control sexual impulses. Either way, this situation will only get more extreme if not dealt with. Please consider telling someone you feel you can trust and begin the process of getting your life back. Too much of a good thing can be too much.

Before you tell, ask yourself why you want to "come out." If you are planning on living full-time in your new gender role, then the need to tell them will be unavoidable. If this is a part-time expression (i.e., cross-dressing) you will have more options on who and when to tell.

What are your motives? *(Ask yourself the following)*

1. Do I want to "shock" them to illicit a reaction?

2. Am I telling them only so my life will be more convenient?
3. Am I hoping to distance myself from them? (i.e., If you wish to leave your wife, but want to shift blame onto her by saying, "Hey I was honest, but she was not accepting.")
4. Am I more excited about my new found freedom or path than how they will feel about it?
5. Do they really need to know about my gender identity issues?
6. Will it improve or degrade my relationship?
7. How old are they, and will the information hurt them needlessly, or do they absolutely have to know?
8. Am I trying to make it easier on them or on me?
9. How much should I tell?
10. Do they have a context in which to understand my words and feelings?
11. Do I wish to be honest and open?
12. Am I planning on blaming them for my "condition?"
13. Am I in a rush? If so, why?

If you answered "yes" to questions 1-4 then you seriously need to rethink your motives. Chances are you have other issues that need to be addressed first, before you "tell all." If you want to shock, damage, or pay back someone by upsetting them with this news, then you should consider repairing the relationship first. If the relationship is over and you need to move on, then state your reasons clearly to them as to why you wish to end your relationship. Do not allow your cross-dressing to become a lightning rod for your relationship-frustrations.

You need to sort out where your impulses are coming from. If this is just a sexual impulse, then you may want to address that reason first. Do you have a lack of intimacy with your spouse or significant other? Would you like to increase your intimacy? Perhaps you should address that first by seeking out a sex therapist, or just have a heartfelt conversation and clear declaration of your needs with your spouse or significant other.

Make sure your motives are sound, and the information you plan to share is within a context that is understandable. Try to put yourself in the shoes of that person and give only the information they are able to understand

and absorb. Speak slowly and let them process what you are saying. Most people can relate to personal feelings. Most family members will listen to you if you talk about cross-dressing and gender identity in terms of your struggle. You can connect on feelings more easily than you can on clinical, medical or scriptural information.

You do not have to tell everything all at once; you can take your time. If they have questions for you, take your time and think about your answers.

Have realistic expectations. Don't assume you will be vilified, nor should you assume that they will fully accept what you are saying. Your guess at how they will respond could be right on or way off. Prepare yourself for the worst case scenario, if possible, but hope for the best.

If you plan on telling your spouse and your relationship is solid, chances are they will be more accepting or empathetic than not. If your marriage is rocky already, the news you are transgender or a cross-dresser usually will not go over well. It could be the "last straw" and become the focal point of an already poor relationship. If your relationships are sound now, chances are this new information will be within the context of a good relationship. If not, the information will just be added to their "list" of why your relationship isn't working. So try and shorten the "list" before you tell them.

The best time to tell is when nothing else is happening. Don't tell on anniversaries, birthdays, Christmas, graduations, funerals, weddings or some other special event. Those you are telling will be the least receptive during these times. When you tell, make sure there is lots of time available to talk about it.

Above all give yourself time. If they are upset, let them vent uninterrupted. Remember the response they give first is mostly emotional. Validate their response and let them be emotional. You have had a long time to think about this, and they may be hearing it for the first time.

Consider talking to a therapist first.

A therapist can give you information about what you are going through in a clinical, yet emotionally supportive fashion. Some advocate having a therapist or knowledgeable friend present when you first tell. This may help to make your case, but could have the result of putting your family member or friend in an adversarial role. They may feel teamed up on and will want to defend themselves.

If you tell them on a one-on-one basis (alone), chances are they will have lots of questions for you anyway. After this initial "telling" they may want to seek out a professional or knowledgeable person's opinion. At this point, you can bring in a therapist or recommend a resource to help them understand.

It is best not to start with, "I have a problem." This will send up red flags and couch the information as completely negative. Instead, try saying, "There is something I want to share with you. I know I can talk to you about anything, and you will be supportive." Starting off in this way should help to affirm your relationship and provide a positive context of trust. If the person begins to freak out at this point, chances are they will not be ready to hear the rest of your speech.

Take them through a brief background about your feelings. Discuss your struggles in terms of feelings. If they can see this is important to you and is something you need to share with them, they should be more responsive and ready to listen. They may even feel good that you trust them so much. Focus in on that.

You will not be able to control the reaction of others, but there are things you can do to help create the best scenario possible. Don't be afraid to share your emotions and let them in.

Although we hopefully have given you some good advice, the response to "telling" is extremely varied. Some will be understanding or even supportive, while others will totally reject the information and perhaps even you. A relationship can become deeper and more fulfilling as a result, or it may end. There are no guarantees. If you are considering telling and decide you really want or need to, then count the cost first and decide if you are willing to pay the price. For many, the freedom and relief in letting someone in is worth the potential backlash.

If the thought of telling is still too scary, start off with a person first who does not impact your life directly. A Stephen Minister at your church perhaps, or a therapist could be a good start. I would not go to your head pastor or deacon first. They have their own agenda and will not usually be concerned with you, but with how this will affect the church congregation. Choose someone you think will be open. Perhaps a clergy from a church in your area that is accepting of those in the LGBTQ community is someone you could talk with or will know of someone. Going it alone is never the optimal choice. You should be able to find someone safe to share this with who will be supportive. There is support for you out there. You are not alone.

Many congregations are becoming aware of transgender issues. As a starting point, here is the web site "Institute for Welcoming Resources," a list of churches that are welcoming to those in the LGBTQI+ community. If one is in your area, they could be a good resource for counseling and affirmation: welcomingresources.org

---

How to Have a Conversation With Your Wife or Partner

There is no single "right way" to approach your spouse.

The first conversation should focus on your story and your feelings. Your story is neither morally wrong nor right. It is simply your story. Your spouse will have very strong feelings about what you are sharing and will need time to process those feelings. Your partner's first reaction will be more emotional than cerebral. Whatever objections you may encounter from family will be fueled by their emotions. If you and your spouse are close, a frank discussion of your feelings (frustrations and struggles) would be best. You have dealt with this for a long time now, and they are more than likely just finding out for the first time. Your first talk should be focused on sharing your feelings.

One way that does not work well, is to "surprise" your family with a presentation of your female alter ego. Don't sit your spouse and the children down in the living room and then disappear for two hours, only to return as "Betty." This is rarely received well. It is best to come out to people one at a time rather than in a group setting.

Try not to be on the defensive or the offensive. It's best to deliver the information from a neutral position. Finger pointing and ultimatums do not work well either.

There are some good clinical resources concerning transgender and gender issues. You might be tempted to plead your case based on those. Clinical information will be helpful down the road, however a clinical dialogue is not the best approach for an initial discussion.

One approach you may want to consider is to open up the topic by asking them if they have ever dealt with gender issues. They may have frustrations with roles at home or on the job. They may want experiences that are normally outside of their cultural gender role. Start your conversation by asking them to share how they feel and then share how you feel.

You have a lot to share, but this "telling" is not about you. It is about them. Start somewhere on common ground and build slowly on that. Give the process some time.

We get our "sense of self" largely from those around us. We rely on the input of others for our identity: How they treat us, how they define us, and if we are accepted or not. We compare and contrast ourselves to others as well: What is their personality compared to ours? What level of education do they have compared to us? How does their career compare to ours? What do they look like compared to us? They, in turn, get their "sense of self" through comparisons and contrasts with us.

Someone who changes (even for a time) something as basic as their gender, changes not only how they are perceived, but also how those they are familiar with perceive themselves. A strong negative reaction to your cross-dressing by family, friends and co-workers has a lot to do with how the cross-dressing directly affects their identity.

Before you tell, ask yourself why you want to. If you are planning on living full-time in your new gender-divergent role, then telling them will more than likely be unavoidable. If this is a part-time expression (cross dressing) you will have more options on who to tell and when.

What are your motives? (Ask yourself the following)

1. How much should I tell?

2. Do I want to "shock" them to illicit a reaction?

3. Am I telling them only so my life will be more convenient?

4. Am I hoping to distance myself from them? (i.e., If you wish to leave your wife, but want to shift blame onto her by saying, "Hey I was honest, but she was not accepting.")

5. Am I more excited about my new found freedom or path than how they will feel about me pursuing it?

6. Do they really need to know about my gender identity issues?

7. Will it improve or degrade my relationship?

8. How old are they, and will the information hurt them needlessly, or do they absolutely have to know?

9. Am I trying to make it easier on them or on me?

10. Do they have a context in which to understand my words and feelings?

11. Do I wish to be honest and open?

12. Am I planning on blaming them for my "condition?"

13. Am I in a rush? If so, why?

These questions are important not only to determine if you should tell, but what do you want to achieve by telling. Try to have a clear idea on what you would like to achieve.

How to Have a Conversation With Your Children

The first rule of thumb is, "share - don't scare!"

When you tell someone about your gender identity issues and cross-dressing, (for those who are married with children) the first question they will ask is, "How does your wife feel about it?" Next will be, "How are your children handling it?"

You will very seldom be asked, "How are you handling it?" People are keenly interested in your family, not so much about you. If your wife and children are okay with your cross-dressing then most others will be as well. Even if your family is just barely okay with it, most of those who would try and counsel you away from your gender expression will back off a bit.

It is important to create a context in which your wife and children feel comfortable with your gender identity exploration. Children are mostly interested in themselves. They want to know that Dad will be there for them no matter what. Your children may already know the terms, "transgender" or "cross-dresser," so let them share what they think a person who is transgender or a cross-dresser might look like.

What you need to do first is provide a positive clear context. The information given should be age appropriate and should relate to how they feel. Use words that they can relate to and understand. Talk about your feelings. Ask how they feel now and share with them how you felt at their age. Above all, do not dress in front of them until the context is set. Halloween can be a fun event to take advantage of. The idea of a costume is readily understandable.

A child is able to absorb information in a positive way if they feel safe and secure. Any conversation about cross-dressing or gender identity must begin with them and end with them. This is not about you.

Gender polarity . . . negative female images . . . laughable transgender "role models" . . . unfocused fear of the unknown, are all ingrained in our culture. To remove all these obstacles may seem like a daunting task. But it is not impossible to remove at least some of these barriers, or at least redefine them.

Educating your children will take some time. It could take a few months to prepare them to hear your information. Please be patient. Here are some tips:

1. If you currently use phrases like, "Don't throw like a girl," or "Stop acting like a sissy," stop using them immediately. This creates a negative image of women, and your professed desire to be more like a woman will be viewed as negative as well.

2. Don't use sexist language in your speech. Avoid terms like fireman, or policeman. Use instead the term "person" to help expand the way in which they view gender and gender roles.

3. Discuss the gender spectrum with them. (When you talk to them, get at their eye level. Look them in the eye and talk with confidence. Body language is very important. Try to be comfortable. Don't rush. You may even want to begin after dinner, and while you are eating desert.)

Explain that on one end of the spectrum is the male. On the other end is the female. Use this basic sort of spectrum:

Male 100% . . . . . 50% (balanced) 50% . . . . 100% Female.

Tell them that all of us have both genders in us. Very few people are 100% anything. Ask them if they know anybody who is either 100% male, or 100% female. This will open up a discussion as to what defines a woman and a man. Let them tell you what the differences are. Children are usually very aware of gender roles. Use their information to help define these gender roles. If you get stuck on this, ask them if they know anybody at school who is “all boy” or “all girl.” Then ask them where they would fit on the gender spectrum. Your son may feel compelled to say that he is 100% boy, or your daughter 100% girl. If you think this will happen, tell him first that you are somewhere in the middle. They will want to follow your lead somewhat. (Even if you at this time in your life feel that you are 100% female, you should not say this.) However, some children who identify as gender fluid may say that they are 100% male AND 100% female. There are no wrong answers.

Go back in time and try to relate to them at their current age level. Tell them how you felt when you were their age. Let them know that you often preferred to play with the girls rather than the boys (if that is true).

The point of this exercise is to “relate” to your children, not to show them how different you are.

Share where you fit on the spectrum. Do not go into a lengthy explanation as to why. Just let the information sit out there. Then, ask them where they fit on the spectrum. If they have questions, keep the answers about yourself brief. Feel free, however, to discuss the information about them in length and end the sessions with positive affirmations about what they have told you. For them to admit this to you, is not unlike your coming out to them. This is risky for them and you need to affirm your acceptance of them. Make this about them first, and about you last.

As time goes on, try to bring up this idea of the gender spectrum as it relates to others. Talk about those you see on TV or around town. Say something like, “Now he is 100% boy.” -or- “I would guess that they are 50-50.” You might even make a game of it.

4. Continue the dialog. Children are mostly interested in how things affect them. Ask them how they feel about themselves. Are they doing well in school? How are their friends treating them? Do they feel like they fit in? Share how you felt in school and some of the problems you had. Tell them a story about your past. Tell it from the perspective of someone who is their age. Talk mostly about your feelings. Ask them if they ever feel this way. Children know that feelings are neither wrong or right.

5. Look for opportunities to affirm those in untypical gender roles. Identify women in roles that are typically male and men in roles that are typically female. Dignify the typical role of a woman as much as you can. Tell them about women you respect and why.

6. Be their friend. Let them in on your life. Tell them what you are doing and why you are interested in it.

7. Do this for several months. The objective is to try to “deprogram” them in how our society has trained them.

8. Dress up for Halloween, or a costume party of some sort. Have FUN with it. Let them help you (if you feel comfortable with that). Talk about how fun this is, and that you enjoy being someone different. Ask who they would like to be, if they could be someone else. Take advantage of this holiday, it is a real gift.

9. Talk about how much you enjoyed your time during Halloween. Tell them that you sometimes have other opportunities to dress up and go out, and that it is a lot of fun. Keep it positive and light-hearted. No details need be given.

10. Ask them if they have any “other identities” that they use. What is the name that they use when they are online? They may hesitate, but let them answer. Most children have some sort of name that they use when playing online games, or that they use as a password, or as an email name. Ask them why they use that name. Share your fem-name with them and tell them how you use it. Don’t be afraid of this. Make it age specific in terms of how you relate this to them. It can be as simple as, “Sometimes people call me Betty.”

11. Let them get used to these ideas. Let these ideas become commonplace. Hint at the fact that you have been working on your female persona, and you are getting much better at it. You will have to show them someday. Wear some gender neutral clothing around the house if you can. DO NOT WEAR YOUR WIFE’S CLOTHING! Children will think that is weird.

12. Involve them in your gender exploration, in a non-threatening manner. If you are honest with them, there is a greater chance that they will be more honest with you when they have issues of their own to share.

Please Consider:

1. Don’t give too much information all at once. Remember, they are only interested in how it affects them. Keep it light-hearted and short. Children may give you support, but do not come to them looking for it, nor should you solicit it.

2. Avoid unwanted discovery. It is best to inform rather than be discovered.

Having a child "find" pictures or emails is rarely ever good. It is best to show them information and explain it in a non-threatening way.

3. Don't be selfish. Children need to feel safe. Make sure that they know they are loved.

4. Remind them about confidences. It is important, within a family, to feel safe and so some of the things we tell each other are just for the family to know. Do not use the word "secret," it carries with it the idea of shame. However, if they do tell their friends, usually this will be a positive thing, because your children will present it in a positive light.

5. Never panic. When someone learns of your T-nature, just smile and share with enthusiasm your freedom and interest.

6. Don't shock. Gathering the family together for a general announcement is fatal 99% of the time. Having "Bernie" disappear for two hours only to come back as "Bernice" is a terrible way to confront your loved ones with this important news. It is lazy and selfish. If you wish to do this, Jerry Springer will be glad to book you.

7. Don't wait to begin. Even if you do not plan on telling your children directly, making them aware of gender issues is a positive step. Begin by giving them information now and reinforce that information when you can. If they end up "finding out" information on your CDing by accident, they will have a good framework established in which to understand and process it.

Short Answers to Long Questions

The questions below are actual questions asked LITC by those in the transgender community. They are unedited and left as asked. These are real concerns from those who find themselves questioning the validity of their desire to express the gender they feel is authentic for them. The responses given address those concerns. LITC helps to answer concerns that hold back some from an honest, healthy gender exploration.

Isn't transgender behavior a mental illness and isn't it related to other "deviant" sexual behaviors?

No to both. Transgender, by itself is an identity and not an illness — mental or otherwise. Years ago it was believed that those identifying as transgender were suffering from multi-personality disorder or schizophrenia. The medical community has in large part recanted that interpretation. Most now hold that the behavior is an expression of gender identity and is akin to having blue eyes.

Some transgender do deal with Gender Identity Disorder (GID) but not all. This diagnosis is used when a person struggles with their gender and has not as of yet self-identified. This condition is considered a disorder, but treated as separate from sexual behavior or orientation. For many transgender, their gender is fluid and not limited to a single expression.

Transgender are NOT sexual deviants. Their gender condition is unconnected to child molestation or any other sexual behavior, coercive or non-coercive. All sexual behaviors statistically cut across all aspects of society, and transgender do not bend the curve one way or the other. Even so, many in American society wrongly view any gender expression that is not strictly mainstream to be "deviant."

Why do I indulge myself in cross-dressing and then purge (throw out all my female belongs)?

This is a common practice among cross-dressers, especially Christian men. Our culture often sees the genders as strictly polarized; male and female. The act of cross-dressing violates and calls into question that gender model. A person may purge their fem items out of a real desire to quit because they see it as culturally wrong or religiously sinful.

Although some freedom exists today to explore actions, dress and mannerisms outside of your gender (more so for females than males) these cross-gender actions are still viewed as outside of what is culturally proper.

Worry over imminent discovery can lead to purging as well. Actual discovery and confrontation will almost always lead to purging.

The cross-dressing experience often is linked to sexual gratification and a desire to stop the sexual activity may lead to purging. Simply saying "no" however and purging rarely addresses the emotional and physical needs that are behind cross-dressing.

The cross-dresser usually has a gender identity issue, or an unresolved psychological or abuse issue that remains even after a commitment is made to cease the actions of cross-dressing. It is important to talk these feelings out. They are difficult to address on your own and you should consider the help of a therapist.

Why do I need to look for affirmation from others and why do I not trust it when I get it?

We are social beings, and have a strong need to belong. It is important to be affirmed in who you are inside, what you look like outside, and what you do. This need is universal. Those who cross-dress often have a low self-image, and are desperate to find affirmation to offset their negative feelings.

Unfortunately, since those who are closeted hide so much of themselves from the world, they may never feel as if they are fully accepted. They believe since no one really knows them, they can never fully trust the positive affirmations of others. Compliments are often discarded because they feel if the person knew the "real me" they would not be so accepting. This is why it is so important to find at least a couple of people who are accepting and you can trust to disclose your gender issues to.

What's the difference between acceptance and tolerance?

Some people may be able to tolerate your cross-dressing, while others will either accept it or be offended by it. To tolerate someone is not the same as accepting them. Those who tolerate are simply keeping their opinions to themselves, but still disapprove of or even hate the individual.

Tolerance is just a staging area for disapproval. Those who tolerate others are not living the Christian model of love. Those who look for the good in others and practice acceptance are pursuing true Christ-like love.

Why do I feel like the "other" gender?

There are many reasons why a person will feel like the opposite gender. Our culture sends out hundreds of gender-biased messages everyday regarding everything we do. This includes judgments and feedback on who we befriend, what job we pursue, what colors we like, what foods we eat, what sports interest us, how we walk, the tone and volume of our voice, where we shop, what we wear, how we argue, what we think is important, and almost everything else we do. Almost every aspect of our lives is defined or quantified by our gender.

It is extremely difficult, if not impossible, to think outside of this two-gender construct. As a result, if a person feels that they are more closely aligned to the gender opposite their birth-gender, that person is painfully aware that they do not fit in.

Since the disapproval they feel from others, or the restrictions that are placed on them are associated with their legal birth gender, they will tend to dislike or reject their legal birth gender in favor of the other gender. This gender confusion can be both physical and psychological.

The gender dysphoria you may be experiencing comes from the incongruity between how you feel inside and what is expected of you based on your legal birth gender. A therapist may be able to help you sort this out.

No matter how much I try to explain how I feel, why do so few people understand?

No one fully understands what is in the mind of another person.

We live our lives with a variety of cultural presuppositions. The way we function and relate to others always revolves around our gender. Much of this we are unaware of because it so completely saturates who we are and how we are treated. When you tell someone else what you are going through, and they do not share in your experience, they will have a difficult time understanding what you are trying to convey because they have no frame of reference.

The best way to communicate is to take time. Look for common ground and find something that you both can relate to and build on that. For example, if you have a child who is into drama you can talk to them about how fun it is to be someone one else sometimes. You can talk about acting and dressing up like someone else. Try to relate to others based on their understanding and life experience.

Why am I so preoccupied with questioning my gender role? Is it unusual to be so aware of my gender?

When we are born, the doctor declares either, “It’s a boy” or “It’s a girl!” It is rare to hear, “It’s a ?????!” The fact that we do not readily allow for alternatives to girl and boy is very telling. Our western society demonstrates a lack of acceptance of those outside the gender norms.

Most people live their whole lives secure in the knowledge they are either a boy or a girl. It defines all that they do. Because it is so ingrained in them, they never question it. It is like breathing the air. We can stop and think about taking a breath but then we go back to being unaware of every breath. A person only becomes aware of their breathing when it becomes difficult or labored.

For those who question their gender identity, each moment is labored. The person who is constantly aware of their gender quantifies even the smallest action as either male or female. They are aware of how they sit, hold their hands, how long their nails are, how big their feet are, what sort of sports interest them, how they cross their legs, and almost everything else.

Those who are comfortable with their gender have aligned themselves culturally with what is expected and so rarely think about gender.

If you find yourself constantly aware of your gender, there is a good chance you have a gender identity issue.

What is this fascination with woman's clothing?

You have heard it said that "clothes make the man," in this case clothes also make the woman. Males and females have different roles in our society. We relate to males and females differently. These gender-based roles are very rigid. Men especially are asked to "be men." If we show a preference or an inclination to enjoy things or activities outside of our assigned gender role we are told emphatically to cease.

Young boys, who in any way act like a girl, are bullied and harassed until they recant. We learn from an early age to hide this part of ourselves or repress these feminine desires, actions and needs. Since we have been brainwashed into thinking only girls are allowed to act and feel the way we do. So if we desire to express ourselves as female, the best way to give ourselves permission to act female is to look female.

One of the biggest thrills for those who cross-dress due to gender identity, is to be treated as female when out in public. The physical pleasure of the clothing is second to that.

For those who cross-dress as a way to work out past abuse or other issues, the clothing itself could be the primary reason. For example, those who have a foot fetish might be into shoes to help them work out some issue in their past. In any case the experience is both physical and psychological and the two together make the desire to cross-dress very compelling.

People who cross-dress do so to allow themselves the freedom to explore more of their inherent personality, interests and issues.

Do I really want to be the opposite gender or is this just some perverted fantasy I am having?

This is a question best answered individually. If you ask this question, more than likely the answer is a bit of both. Each person needs to ascertain what part of the expression is natural and healthy and which part is harmful. If by perverted you mean, lots of casual, or sexual torture, then those could be symptoms of other issues you need to take care of.

If you are calling cross-dressing itself perverted simply because you are ashamed of it, then you need to find away to deal with the shame. Ask yourself what part of cross-dressing are you ashamed of? Why are you ashamed of it? You may have other issues that need to be addressed.

Those who cross-dress often have gender issues they need to work out.

Am I just being selfish? Why do I put my obsession with cross-dressing over my family and those I love?

The act of cross-dressing is by its nature a selfish act in that it is something you do for yourself. Exercise could be a selfish act. Any hobby or past time that benefits only you could be a selfish act. The question, "Is it selfish," begs the question, "Do you think you are worth spending personal time on?" If you were suffering from cancer, would spending time receiving radiation treatments be considered selfish? I firmly believe that you need to take care of yourself to be a better person for your family and relations.

If you do not take care of your needs and desires (at least to some extent) you more than likely will be difficult to live with and eventually get very depressed. How is that being a good husband, father, employee or caregiver? When the oxygen mask drops from the top of the airplane the instructions say to put yours on first and then help the person next to you. If you are depleted and depressed and just staying afloat, you need to take care of yourself, and put yourself in a good frame of mind to be able to be there for others.

So many intelligent people that I respect say I am sinning. Are they right?

Maybe they are, and maybe they aren't. If someone insists on labeling an action as sinful, then there needs to be an understanding of what sin is. The Bible says that even our righteousness is like filthy rags compared to the grace of God. Do you think that any action, including cross-dressing, is exempt from this? Everything we do has an element of "sin" attached to it when sin is defined as imperfection. We never have purely godly motives; it is not in our nature. Those who think they are close to being sin-free understand neither grace nor the glory that is God. God tells us to use sober judgment when we think of ourselves. In the light of God's glory, we are the lost sheep, we are the missing coin, we are the prodigal son.

If you are drowning and someone tries to "help" you, do they bring a life preserver or a heavy stone? Is a person hiding rocks in their hands while they talk to you, or are their hands open ready to give you a hug? Those who focus in on the sins of others do so to avoid their own failings. Those people you respect may be knowledgeable about many things; however cross-dressing may not be one of them. Asking, "Is it a sin," is not really the most important question to ask.

The best course of action is not to try and justify your actions, but to be honest about them, at least with yourself. God already knows your heart, better then you do, and for those who (even in a small way) want to be his child, he has a gold ring, a fine garment, and an everlasting hug.

If being transgender is so prevalent then why is the medical community only just now addressing it? What research is being done?

Historically there has been, in the US, a cultural resistance to the idea that there could be a third, fourth or fifth gender. As a result, much of the information and validity for a third, fourth or fifth gender model has not been pursued.

It may seem like the medical community is only now addressing gender identity, but that is not true. Historically there have always been some in the medical community that have researched gender and gender, affirming medical procedures. In recent years, there has been more of a concerted effort to address gender issues.

The medical community for the most part deals with illnesses and the treatment of illnesses. Wellness care is only recently been addressed for those who identify as transgender, and those who are part of the larger gender spectrum. Many medical associations have established standards of care for transgender and non-binary persons.

For better or worse, the condition known as *gender identity disorder* was pronounced as a disorder so that the medical community could bring it under its umbrella of care and so it would be covered by health insurance. If the condition of gender identity disorder were not a disorder, they would not be able to treat it. Basically, unless you are sick or broken, they do not address your health issues. Gender Identity Disorder is considered an undesirable condition because the medical community promotes the idea that there are two and only two genders. The research currently is geared towards cause and cure.

Very little research is being done by the medical community that calls into question the validity of the Western culture's two-gender model. It still remains as the norm. Even so, there are some advances that have expanded the concepts of male and female.

Google it! There is a wave of research that has been forming and continues to expand the care for those dealing with gender identity.

Glossary of Terms

Androgen

A generic term for any natural or synthetic compound, usually a steroid hormone, that stimulates or controls the development and maintenance of masculine characteristics by binding to androgen receptors. This includes the activity of the accessory male sex organs and development of male secondary sex characteristics. Androgens, which were first discovered in 1936, are also called androgenic hormones or testoids. The most well-known androgen is testosterone.

Androgynes

A person who is psychologically androgynous. The word androgyne was previously applied only to androgynous floral. The word is now being used to describe the personhood of an androgynous individual. This may include a person with an androgynous physical appearance, a person with a combination of both masculine and feminine personality traits, or a person who has no sense of being either male or female. Not everyone who is androgynous looking is an androgyne, and not every androgyne looks androgynous.

Androgenous

A person who dresses in a non-specific gender fashion. Being both male and female or neither. Presenting as neither clearly masculine or feminine. Having an ambiguous sexual or gender identity. Being both male and female; hermaphrodite.

Andropause

The impact of decreasing androgens is known as andropause, also called "male menopause" or PADAM – Partial Androgen Deficiency in the Aging Male. It is a normal part of aging, although, for some men it is accompanied by a gradual and undesired decline in their sexuality, mood and overall energy. Sometimes it can even expose men to more serious health risks. Basically, testosterone levels drop while estrogen percentages increase.

Legal Birth Gender

The gender assigned to a person at birth. This usually relates to the genitalia that are the most prominent. All babies have the potential for either gender when they are first conceived. A combination of hormones and genetics can create a wide range of gender expressions. Sometimes the genders are ambiguous and the doctors and parents will often promote one gender over through the use of surgery and or hormones. A large number of babies are born inter-sexed but even so will often be raised as a specific gender. This is not true in every culture, but in the Western culture we hold to a very rigid male and female only gender model. Children are normally asked to choose between the two.

Cross-dress

Dressing in the manner of the opposite gender.

Cross-dressing (Cross-dressing or cross dressing)

The act of wearing clothing normally associated with the other gender. There are a variety of reasons for cross-dressing. Most have to do with gender identity, but there are many other reasons as well. Normally there is a distinction made between someone who is a cross-dresser and someone who is transgender. Referring to a transgender person as "just a cross-dresser" is often regarded as demeaning or insulting.

Cross-dressers (cross-dressers or cross dressers)

Those who wear the clothing of the "other" gender but have little desire to physically alter their gender. The reasons and catalysts to cross-dress are varied. It may result from fundamental brain chemistry, reconciling abuse from a parent or trusted caregiver (usually resulting in a fetish), biologically inter-sexed, or simple curiosity. Often cross-dressing is done for comfort or to relieve tension, and usually has a sexual component attached to it.

Cross-Gender

When a person expresses themselves in a manner related to the other gender. This includes cross-dressing, mannerisms, interests, choice of friends, career and any other function that relates to a specific gender. The notion that someone has crossed a gender line stems from the idea that the polarized gender model contains gender dictums that cover a wide range of actions and activities.

Drab

When a person dresses as their legal birth gender. This term is usually used when a cross-dressing male is not presenting as female, but as a male. Also used to signify the dress-code for a particular outing or event. ie:"Come in drab that day."

Dressed

When a person dresses as the other gender.

Drag Queens or Drag Kings

These individuals usually dress as an iconic gender image simply for fun. This group is the one most people see on the news and on stage. Most of those engaged in this activity are part of the LGBTQI+ community, however, anyone dressed as an exaggerated gender stereotype would qualify.

Enfemme

A man who dresses up as a woman, or a boy who dresses up as a girl for the purpose of acting or living as a person of that gender. Enfemme or En-femme refers to the exhibiting a female presentation by a male. Dressing as completely female in order to pass as a female is referred to as full-enfemme.

Eunuch

A person who is of the third gender (or sex). Many were born this way, however in ancient times infants were often castrated early to stop the hormonal changes and make a male more feminine or gender neutral. These individuals were then employed in a variety of services. The most well-known being that of harem servants. Many were employed as domestics, religious specialists, servants of the ruler, or even military commanders. According to Byzantine historian Kathryn Ringrose, while the pagans of Classical Antiquity based their notions of gender purely on the physical, the Byzantine Christian based their definitions of gender more on the behavior of the person. More about eunuchs may be found at the following link.

For more information: http://en.wikipedia.org/wiki/Eunuch

F2M

Female to male transgender. Someone who is born biologically female but identifies as male, and will usually present as male.

Gender Blessed

When a person exhibits the traits and actions of both genders, and feels comfortable in either role to some extent, they are known as gender blessed. This label is used in contrast to the term gender identity disorder in that the condition of being transgender is look at as a positive state rather than a negative one. (See two-spirits.)

Gender-Congruent

A harmonious balance of physical gender and psychological gender identity (gender-congruency).

Gender-Divergent

To deviate from a person's assigned biological legal birth gender. Becoming different in form or kind. To depart from the gender that society has labeled you (gender-divergence).

Gender Dysphoria

Being discontented with the biological legal birth gender. A term to describe the separation between a person's psychological, emotional and biological genders.

Gender Euphoria

The act of cross-dressing may cause the brain to release endorphins. This intense elation is known as gender euphoria. This euphoria is usually experienced the first few times a person cross-dresses, but may be felt each time a person is dressed and last for years until the newness wears thin.

Gender Fluid

Most who define themselves as gender fluid, do so by expressing both of the gender binaries of male and female, as well as the non-binary at different times. The way this is expressed differs from person to person. Many trans youth have embraced this identity since it can be appropriated uniquely. This term was first introduced by Kate Bornstein, author of Gender Outlaw, and later mainstreamed into Western Culture at the 2010 Transgender Religious Leaders Summit in Berkeley California by Minister Kathy Randall Klein, Rev. Megan Rohrer, Rev. Louis Mitchell, and Chris Paige MDiv. The term was promoted on the Light in the Closet website as well as the Gender Tree website, authored by Sandra Stewart.

Gender-Incongruent

A psychological state where physical gender and psychological gender are out-of-sync (gender-incongruency).

Gender Linked

When actions are based on gender, and viewed as either appropriate or not. Actions, thoughts and expressions may be acceptable or expected from one gender and not the other. This is associated with the polarized two-gender model of male and female.

Gender Variance

A term that refers to those expressions of gender that do not conform to the dominant gender norms (masculinity and femininity) of Western culture.

Gender Queer and Inter Gender

These are terms for gender identities other than man or woman. People who identify as gender queer may think of themselves as being both genders rather than choosing either male or female. They have embraced a gender identity well outside of the polarized gender model of male and female. Some see "gender queer" as a third gender to complement the traditional two, while others identify as genderless or a-gender. Gender queer can also be an umbrella term for the queer community

Inter-Sexed or Hermaphrodites

Many people are born with genitals which show characteristics of both genders. Most have surgery while they are still infants. In the last few years though, the validity of this early surgery has come into serious questioning, mostly due to the fact that those who have been subjected to this alteration often feel they grew up with an essential part of themselves missing. A term also used is third gender.

LGBT (also GLBT/GLBTI/LGBTQI+/LGBTQI)

LGBT is an initialism referring to Lesbian, Gay, Bisexual and Transgender/ transsexual people. This term was first used in the 1990s. GLBT is also used, but with the terms in a different order. GLBTI has added an additional term or group, "Inter-sexed" as well. GLBTI is fairly new, and reflects an attitude of allowing for additional gender expressions. Sometimes the letter "S" is added as well to include the term "Straight." LGBTQI+ adds the category of Gender Queer.

M2F

Male to female transgender. Someone who is born biologically male but identifies as female. They usually present as female.

Opposite Gender

There are many causes and catalysts that would make an individual desire to become more like the "opposite gender." Even in writing this I hesitate to use the term "opposite gender" for that implies a strictly polarized gender model. I use this term only to communicate a starting point in which to understand the concepts of male and female.

Purge

Throwing out all your cross-dressing items, clothing, make-up, etc. This usually takes place after the person who cross-dresses experiences guilt, and has determined never to cross-dress again.

Purging Cycle

A man or woman who cross-dress, then throws out all his feminine items away, or her masculine items, only to purchase more. Cross-dresses again and then throws it all away again. This cycle may continue over and over for years.

Polarized Gender Model (also known as bi-gender or two-gender)

In most Western cultures, genders are seen as only two; male and female. Some cultures recognize three genders and others even five, seven or over fifty. Our mainstream Western culture however adheres to a rigid two gender model, although this is now being challenged. As a result, those who feel like they are both genders, somewhere in-between, or neither male or female, find themselves often relegated to one polarized gender or the other. Our Western culture does not readily dignify those who are outside of this polarized gender model. The Western culture, in practicality, is so fixed on the idea of just two genders that any expression outside of your assigned gender is looked upon disapprovingly.

Third Gender

Also known as third sex. These are individuals that are neither defined as men nor women. Some societies recognize three or more genders. The state of being neither strictly male nor female is in relation to their biology, but can also apply to the spirit or psychology of the person. A person may experience gender identity disorder as a result, however most in this third gender do not view themselves as deficient or broken. More information can be found visiting the web site below.

For more information: http://en.wikipedia.org/wiki/Third_gender

Transgender / Trans

Often used as an umbrella term for any person who bends the so-called traditional gender roles. Primarily applied to individuals whose gender identity is skewed towards the gender opposite their assigned legal birth gender. They may identify in part or in full with this other gender. Included are cross-dressers, transsexuals, transgenderist and androgynes. Some transgender dress in a non-specific or androgynous gender fashion. Most transgender express this gender identity by wearing clothing that is associated with the other gender and participate in social activities typical for the person of that gender. Many individuals simply identify as transgender without citing a specific sub-category or expression.

Those who struggle with something as fundamental as gender often find themselves also dealing with social stigma or isolation. Many find themselves outside of society, and so seek out other transgender and form communities of their own.

Being a trans person is not a matter of sexual orientation. Often a person who is transgender is mis-labeled as a person who is homosexual. Not all trans people identify as part of the GLB community but some do. The percentage of transgender who identify as homosexual is about the same as the general population.

Although being transgender is not directly related to a person's sexual orientation or sexual activity, much of the information found on the Internet is skewed towards sex and pornography (there is big money in pornography, not so much money in dispensing clinical information).

While a person's sexual impulses and orientation are related to gender, the issue of gender identity is distinct from the issue of sexuality. People are sexual beings regardless of gender identity and those impulses exist regardless. It is important to have a discussion about gender that is separate from sexual drives.

The word trans is a shorter version of transgender and more often used now. It is usually used when identifying a specific gender such as, "trans man" and "trans woman" or identifying an age group such as "trans youth:"

Transgenderist

This term is used infrequently to describe a person who lives as a member of the opposite gender either fulltime or part-time, but are not pursuing sexual reassignment. This choice is not by default but rather a conscious decision. They may have facial reconstruction, breast implants and take other measures to look like the other gender, but stop short of sexual reassignment. Sometimes referred to as shemales in the porn industry. (Shemale is consider by most a disrespectful term and invalidates the life choice.) Some who cross-dress prefer to apply the term transgenderist to themselves to allude to their gender-divergent identity and heterosexuality. This term is more narrow in its focus than the more general term transgender.

Transsexual

People who desire to change their gender by fundamentally altering their bodies in order to live as members of the "other" gender. This is accomplished through surgical procedures, hormones, and other medical technologies and may or may not include genitalia sexual reassignment. The issue of sexual gratification is separate from gender identity, as is the issue of sexual orientation.

Transvestite

An older term that refers to a person (especially a male) who adopts the dress and often the behavior typical of the opposite gender, especially for purposes of emotional or sexual gratification. Also known as Tranny.

They / Their / Them (non-specific gender form in place of he/she)

These words have been used for decades when a person is unsure of a another's gender. When you do not readily identify a gender, someone may say, *"I think I saw them jump over the fence. I do not know what they were doing."* In this case an individual has been identified in the neutral as a single person.

These terms may be used without defining one as male or female. Also used by a person who self-defines as neither the male nor female gender. "They, them, theirs" are often used as pronouns.

"They" is used as a singular-plural word within the context of a sentence instead of the clumsily he/she. The term he/she alludes to a strict interpretation of the polarized gender model and does not allow for those who are transgender, gender queer, inter-sexed or hermaphrodites.

There have been attempts to create new terms, but instead it is reasonable to use existing language within this context and broaden the application of the words "they, their, them and themselves." In the context of he/she, the word they is the nominative case form (singular or plural within the context), them the objective, their the possessive, and themselves the intensive and reflective. - n. pl. they're a person.

Two-Spirits

In some ancient cultures as with many of the native American tribes, those who were born exhibiting traits that would define them as transgender, or those who were biologically inter-sexed or gender nonspecific were known as two-spirits. These individuals were highly valued and were often encouraged to be medicine men, shamen or counselors.

Coined in 1990, Two-Spirit is a modern, pan-Indigenous umbrella term specific to North American Native cultures, but similar third-gender and gender-diverse roles exist in many different cultures globally.

NOTE: This list of terms is not an exhaustive list, and we apologize if some of the definitions are not more extensive or incomplete. Language is dynamic and definitions change constantly. This list was intended to give a brief understanding of some basic terms. Any omissions are unintentional and not purposefully excluded.

Who am I?

The story of a trans youth.

This story is an autobiographical account of a trans youth. Growing up with GID is difficult and fitting in with peers hard. This story is not uncommon.

Introduction:

I was a child.

The joy of my day was defined by new discoveries fresh and sweet. Feelings were neither wrong nor right but just experienced. It was only later that those feelings were defined for me, by either a gold star on the corner of lined yellow paper or the taste of Ivory soap.

I clearly remember many yesterdays. Some of them fondly, others with heart-wrenching pain and salty tears. All of them blend together to form my life. The happy times harvest a reward unto themselves. The amusement park rides, and presents on Christmas morning are reminisced through a fuzzy filtered lens, both soft and kind.

The difficult times, however, glean something better. There is a purity of thought and emotion that can only be achieved when stumbling through the fiery furnace of adversity. The insights inherent to this process usually flower over time. Difficulties experienced are what define my character and mold my perception of the path on which I journey. The joys that are birthed through fire are more akin to the safe warmth of an old sweater than the elation of a roller coaster ride.

Chapter One: School Rules

A red rubber playground ball thumps a hollow twang that is immediately echoed by the clank of a recess line-up bell. Sounding more like a broken alarm clock, the chime rings out the one-minute warning. I race past my 6-year-old-peers to get to the front of the line. We had to line up for everything; entering and exiting the brown and beige colored classrooms for breaks, getting food at the cafeteria, and finally waiting to board the yellow school bus that would take us home. (I loathe lines to this day.) I am met this time by a grumpy volunteer mom who reminds me in a rather coarse voice that "ladies" go first. She tells me to be polite and stand aside. I wait as the parade of pink, soft blue and purple dresses queue up in front of me.

"Girls first?" I thought. "I wish I were a girl, then I could go first." I mulled over what life would be like as a girl. Lining up as requested, I follow my classmates into room "2." The smell of stale chalk and paper greet me as I am herded past our teacher, Mrs. Gunder, into my stall. Still, I couldn't shake the thought. "I wish I were a girl..." The sentence reverberated in my mind. I fantasized about it during the rest of the day.

I went home and played that night with my sister and her dolls.

As the weeks and months went by, I still could not shake the thought. "I wish I were a girl". Even after that ridiculous "girls first" rule became politically incorrect the thought remained and grew stronger.

My younger sister of two years loved me, her big brother. I was creative and inventive. We would play dress-up together, she would squeal in delight at my interest. My older brother laughed at this exercise as only an older sibling could. So I played dress-up when he wasn't around. One of my favorite games was to take the heads off "Barbie" and "Ken" and switch them. They never quite fit right. But I attempted it often. GI Joe fit better but the result was rather disturbing.

I went through many male playmates. I never seemed to hold onto those relationships as easily as I could the girls I considered to be friends. I didn't know why. It seemed like I just wore them out. When I tried to get "into" a group of my male peers, I found it rather confusing and lonely.

On a sunny Friday afternoon, during forth grade, I began to become aware that something was wrong. I tried hard to fit in, by just being myself. But a lot of the guy talk I found offensive. My saving grace was church and playing sports. People who you admired in the classroom could be on the same team as you and you both would for a brief time be working for a common goal. A form of temporary friendship. I loved the competition and wished the games could go on forever. I thought I was pretty good too, but this assessment was not shared by my peers especially when it came time to pick teams.

Usually Dave and Bob were the team captains. They were the biggest and fastest, so we naturally, deferred to their wisdom.

Dave would always pick Brian first (his best friend).

Bob was a little more democratic and not always so predictable, he chose Paul this time.

Dave looked right at me and then asked for "Mike."

Bob thought carefully as we, the remaining 6 applicants, all shuffled our feet and tried to look cool. "I'll take Mark."

Dave quickly fired back, "Joe." Joe didn't move.

"My name is Joseph, not Joe." he said deliberately. He reminded us of the distinction on a daily basis, but at least no one ever called him Joey. The proper correction made, he too took his place.

Bob countered with, "Raymond" (clear to all a better choice than Joe).

Only three spots left and four "want-to-plays". I would be sure to go soon. After all I was well rested. I hadn't been picked all week. Hey... look at me... fresh legs!

Dave started to speak, hesitated, then paused and thought hard. The universal signs that the pickings had gotten pretty slim. I guess I'll take "Peter."

Now I was getting nervous. Me, little Mike and Doug started to plead our case with winning looks. Dave never chose me and it was Bob's turn. I did the math. If I didn't go this round I would be out again. Would Bob pick Doug? No, Doug was terrible. He was big, but slow and not real bright. This year I was slightly taller than little Mike, so maybe I would have the advantage. Mike and I compared our heights to each other at regular intervals. One of us was always the shortest in the class, depending on who had the latest "growth spurt." It had been that way all throughout Elementary school.

I liked Bob, he was thoughtful. He looked at me and then Little Mike and glanced over at Doug. The three of us could hardly contain our anxiety. Pick me, pick me our bodies screamed! He turned and looked Dave straight in the eye. Then he broke with tradition, "You can have Doug and I'll take the other two." he suggested. Bob waited quietly for a reply.

Dave was caught off guard. What? Not play with even teams? That was the standard excuse not to get stuck with what was perceived as the weakest player. However, Dave rationalized, "If I don't agree, then Bob will surely pick Doug and I'll get stuck with one of the other two." So he agreed.

Today both "Little Mike" and I were picked. I still thought I should have realistically gone in the third round and I mentioned this to Bob who only smiled back.

Because it was football season that was the sport of the day. With only 20 minutes of recess left, we quickly went to work.

It now started to dawn on Dave that he had fewer players and perhaps had made a fatal error in judgment. So insisted on "us" kicking off to "them."

It was easy to stop their weak attack. Dave usually tried to throw to one of the first two draft picks, so Bob had those players well covered. Bob had both Little Mike and I blitz on the agreed "three alligator" count. This left poor Dave, who always played center, with the task of blocking both of us. We were an unstoppable combination.

On offense, it was a dream come true. Bob did the unexpected and actually used Little Mike and I on pass patterns. Doug was no match for the two of us. I scored three touchdowns and had one interception. It felt better than great. Easily one of my best young moments. I was elated the rest of the day and into the weekend.

The weekend flew by. I could hardly wait till it was time for recess again. I got up Monday morning eager to get to school. I boarded the yellow and black school bus with pride, knowing I was finally viewed by its occupants in the way I should have been all along, the same way I always viewed myself.

Year after year, I was one of the shortest boys in my grade. Even so I did not think myself as radically different or inferior. Quite the opposite. I always had a healthy self-esteem. I knew that God loved me and so did my parents. I was aware that I was short, but I liked it. I liked who I was and didn't wish to be someone else. I knew I was smarter than most of the kids and loved to banter with the teachers about all sorts of topics. I challenged myself with difficult math problems and would draw and color for hours. When I wasn't inventing a new product, I was writing books, jokes and planning out academy award winning screenplays. When I wasn't included in their "reindeer games" I figured it was their loss not mine. They just didn't know what they were missing. I felt like Rudolph on a foggy Christmas Eve.

Today as the bus bounded along the roughly paved roads, all things seemed new. Last Friday I flew on the playground for the first time and all had watched. They finally saw some of my vast hidden potential, tapped into it and I'm sure had marveled at its depth.

We queued up for class and entered the school room, ladies first. As I sat at my desk I became impatient with our instructor Mr. Wallis as he droned on and on about what? Japan and the industrial revolution? What does that have to do with this glorious day? I'm sure he must of heard about my overwhelming victory on the field of honor. I counted the minutes before the next recess.

My mind wondered, "Perhaps I would be picked first." I could see it now. The logic was so obvious. I smiled.

The recess bell never sounded so clear.

We all rushed outside in a hurry to get as much playtime as possible. This was one day I was glad I wasn't ball monitor. Usually I enjoyed being ball monitor. It was a low-key position of authority. I requested the opportunity from Mr. Wallis often. Ball monitor meant you had to wait until all the balls had been taken, or the last student had gone and visa versa at the end of recess. You counted them and marked down who took what. Also the ball monitor got to go into the classroom first, along with the girls.

Today was different. I would be picked first and had to hurry to get out to the field. "C'mon guys, let's play football." I hurried my fellow classmates along as if I had invented the game myself and wanted to show it to them for the first time.

Much too slowly the applicants lined up for the selection process. Bob wasn't here today, so it was agreed that Paul and Dave would be captains.

Dave, as usual, went first and chose Brian. Not a big surprise.

Now I was sure it was my turn. I think I even began to step forward in expectation.

Paul looked right at me and then asked for "Mike."

The rest was like a bad dream. I think I had my first out-of-body experience. The air around me took on a surreal quality. Colors became confused and the world looked twisted, unfamiliar and frightening as one by one players were selected until I was standing, again, alone. As they all walked away, a protest which was churning deep inside my heart vomited forth in a single word. "Stop!" I cried.

As the heaviness in the air cleared I hurried up to Dave. "What's happening here? What happened to last week? I scored, don't you remember?"

Dave was startled. He fumbled for an answer. What he said, I don't remember. I wasn't really listening. It made no sense. It wasn't fair. I had been exposed for the first time to the "Good-ol-boys club" and realized that my membership had been denied. I had won, proven myself worthy. What was the matter? What did they know about me that I didn't?

I enjoyed the company of the girls a lot and would play with them when it was acceptable. I would usually focus in on one male friend at a time. These male relationships usually last about half a school year. I was never sure why they would shy away from me. I found the company of females much more relaxing.

Church was one of my favorite places to go. I loved the bible stories. The weak conquering by the grace of God. Jesus' amazing life quite often confused me, but the discovery of truth, doctrine and the interpretations which followed were a source of revelation and excitement.

I talked to God constantly, he was a source of comfort and extreme joy. Most of my peers wanted to be sports heroes or firemen, I wanted to be a minister. I had declared to my mother at the tender age of four my intentions and had not wavered much since then. Sometimes it was a missionary, or a pastor, and for a while I wanted to be a nun. I really enjoyed the TV series with "Sally Fields." I thought that being able to fly would have been the greatest feeling imaginable. Often I would dream of flying and wake up knowing that if the right conditions existed, I could fly.

Sally Fields really helped fuel my imagination. A small weak woman who loves and serves God, and could fly. Wouldn't that be something? She would use her special powers each week to help others, and also to get some outrageous aerial footage. Forget Bart Star, I'll take Sister Sally Fields. She was easily one of my first crushes. I wanted to know her; I wanted to be her. I freely told others about my love of Sally Fields. I honestly didn't know that my desires were any different that those of the children around me.

Chapter 2: The Fight

It was about a month before graduating from sixth grade. It was a windy day, and we had spent most of the recess holding our coats over our heads like sails and letting the wind blow us around. Don and I were playing jacks with the girls when Dave with a small entourage approached. He walked straight up to me and for a moment I felt honored by the attention. He asked me to stand, and not seeing any reason not to, I complied. He had a funny look on his face and I couldn't read what he was thinking. Just then a couple of his friends pushed Little Mike forward. He forced us back to back and declared it would be a fair fight.

For some reason I would get into a lot of fights. I was often challenged, and never backed down. The competition was exhilarating and the contact not unpleasant. I had a strange sense of humor and my timing often wasn't the best. Usually saying exactly what you think tends to annoy people. And I did so on a daily basis. Here I was again.

The time as usual was after school. The place (surprise, surprise) the baseballs diamond. Oh great -- dirt. Well, I'll just try not to fall this time. My favorite place to fight, however, was the Fire Station. The grass was softer, the field smaller, and exposed to traffic on two sides. Harder to get ganged up on there, and it felt a little more intimate. Besides, medical attention was close by.

School let out, and we all made our way out to the dirt lot. Dave laid down the rules. "No kicking you know where..." he went on with the traditional verbiage for gentlemanly conduct.

I fought a lot, not usually questioning why. Sometimes my friends and I would do so just for the sake of competition.

Dave startled me with what he said next.

"This is to determine who the smallest and the weakest in our class is," he blurted out.

I was about to object, so was Little Mike.

Then he continued, as he fluffed himself up to his height of nearly 6 feet. "Whoever backs out will not be allowed to play with us anymore. He will lose by chickening out." He crowed this out like some red and white-striped carnival ring announcer. The crowd, which had gathered, confessed the inescapable sixth grade logic of the statement with a series of grunts and groans. Heads bobbed up and down and it reminded me of birds floating on the sea being tossed about by waves.

I liked Little Mike. We were not exactly friends, but he was always nice enough. I think we had been good friends once, for the usual 6-month stint. Dave encouraged us not to keep the crowd waiting. If I walked I would be ostracized. I thought I already was in most ways. Seldom did I get to play with them anyway. I think my perspective on life confused them.

This declaration of Dave's seemed to me rather rigid and pointless. Little Mike made the decision clearer by agreeing first. The ball was in my court now, would I chicken out? My possible future success on the playground was inexplicably and irrationally at stake. How was this possible? What or who gave Dave the right to determine, on a whim, our destinies? I suppose we did. The crowd waited.

As was my custom, I would not hit first, so I motioned to Mike if he wanted to start something he would have to throw the first punch. This may sound magnanimous, but I had discovered three things. The first punch is tentative and usually didn't do much damage. Also, you could always claim you were defending yourself (I did not want to get into trouble), and finally, more often than not, it left your opponent wide open to retaliation. His first punch landed on my upper body, I cradled it and returned two swift blows. A right and then left to the face. Little Mike went down and the "fight" was over. The crowed cheered, and I was given the obligatory congratulations by being hoisted up into the air.

This lasted all of a few seconds. My thoughts quickly returned to Little Mike. I hope he wasn't hurt too bad. I went to his house after school to check on him.

Nothing, for either me or Little Mike really changed much. I was glad that I wasn't the tool after all of his official banishment to the world of the un-befriended. As usual, we were still both picked last, if at all. I felt used. I was angry with Dave, but mostly with myself for allowing myself to be goaded into such a pointless and mean-spirited contest. I liked the competition. I didn't like the feelings of shame and remorse. Although I didn't hit the ground, I felt dirtier than Little Mike who had. I determined not to allow myself to be used that way again.

Sixth grade ended, and so my journey into the world of puberty was about to begin. I was actually looking forward to it. Ignorance is, as they say, bliss.

Chapter 3: Experimenting

Okay, so I liked Barbara Streisand. I also loved to watch Sally Fields (who gets better with age) as well as Katherine Hepburn and Audrey Hepburn. I freely offered my opinions, but slowly began to realize that many of my interests were not shared by my male peers.

At this point in my life, I started to become aware of the need for separation. Playing dress-up with my sister stopped, and became something hidden and more personal. The more I suppressed these emotions and desires, the more intense they became. I was not yet (sexually) developed, but from the shore of my childhood I could see the tidal wave approaching. I was unclear what color the water would be.

During the day much of what I did was normal. I was very polite and never swore. I did not rebel and felt sorry for those who did. I had a reputation as being funny, artistic, and very quirky. The girls liked my gentle nature and soft heart. I treasured a deep love of biblical scriptures and freely spoke to others about Jesus Christ. I found friends (many girls), of like mind, and had a very good time.

The playground rules, as known in elementary, disappeared somewhat in intermediate school. There were lots of new faces and most everyone felt a little lost at first. I was however destined to continue some of the same relationships as before. But this time we had a common bond, fear. Fear of the unknown. I began to grow up and so did the attitudes of most of my peers. Many of those same boys who tried to shun me eventually wore down, and I was accepted in the sports arena. We played a lot of street ball and sandlot ball together. I wasn't always picked last, and usually played.

I loved to dance, and even took some classes. My parents were usually very supportive of my interest in art, writing, music and sports.

Our neighborhood had lots of backyard dances. Thank God for Crystal Blue Persuasions. It was a great slow song. It was a safe way for us boys to explore our sexuality with the neighborhood girls.

I finally grew a little and was no longer the absolute shortest. I also stopped measuring completely. It was not relevant. During this time I landed a job, which provided me hours alone by myself in a private home. This provided a venue quite different than any I had experienced.

It was a Monday morning. I had been working for a couple of days previously. My dad pulled his car up to the front of the job sight and dropped me off. I would not picked up until later in the day.

At lunchtime I walked down to a small shopping center to purchase food. I purchased the usual, cold cuts, melted cheese, chips and an orange soda. I sat down outside on the soft grass and leaned back, letting the sun warm me. I then got an impulse. I went next door to the five and dime. The cosmetic counter was full of the missing pieces that could make my transformations more believable: false eyelashes, lipstick, makeup, and stockings. I gathered up my purchases and walked sheepishly up to the counter.

Walking up to the lady in the blue and white checked apron working the cash register, I declared, “It is my sister’s birthday and she is turning 13.” She was actually turning 11, but 13 sounded more plausible. “As a joke I am purchasing some items for her. Do you have any suggestions?”

She looked me up and down.

“Are you sure you’re not purchasing these for yourself?” she questioned.

I laughed. “That’s pretty funny,” I said and then continued. “No, really, any other suggestions?” She helped me pick out a few more items and I left. I couldn’t walk back to the abandoned home fast enough. I wasn’t embarrassed; I was excited.

I experimented with the different items and at home that night snuck back into the bathroom for a more complete look. I really liked what I saw. So much so that I would risk walking around the house at night with the lights off just to feel the air brushing past the skirts and tops and nylons. It was a risk, but the desire to experiment was stronger than the apprehension.

My dress-up sessions had become more frequent. This was probably due to the coming of the aforementioned wave. I would hide my mother’s clothes near my bed and then slip into the bathroom when everyone was asleep. She owned wigs and a whole assortment of boots and jewelry. These made a quick transformation easy. To my later disbelief, I never got caught. I thought they must know, but they didn’t, or decided not to say anything.

At this time, the wave still had not crashed upon the shore. My desire to connect with my feminine side was more innocent than sexual. Although ready for the onslaught, I had not yet developed physically enough to understand the feelings inside, nor fan the pre-puberty embers which were glowing. I just knew for now, it felt right and I was happy.

The innocence I enjoyed in those early days would not last.

Eventually the fear of discovery and the disapproval from the church, school and family would erode away at my opportunities to explore. Although the feelings never lessened, I became well practiced over the years in denying my feminine self and the weight of my secret became unbearably heavy.

High school, college, job, marriage and children were all experienced and took priority. Authentic gender exploration was something I had little time for and I took great pains to ignore, stuff, and conceal it.

I now realize that denying such a large part of myself was both physically and mentally harmful. I was created to be who I am and trying to fit exclusively into a male persona resulted in the loss of my personhood.

It was in my forties that I finally succeeded in shutting that side of my identity down. In doing so, I completely lost myself to such an extent that I could not even recognize my reflection in the mirror.

Although I still had young children, I was exhausted and did not see a way out. It was then that I started to plan a way to leave. I prayed for God to mercifully take me.

As the date of my departure neared, it was my wife who made me face my gender reality and stopped me from pursuing what I felt was an inevitable conclusion. With her support, love and compassion she found avenues for me to explore safely. I sought out other physiological and medical support to understand what I was going through. It took time, but I was able to integrate and appreciate all of who I am.

I had to let go of what I mistakenly thought were my God ordained cultural male expectations. I was reborn into a deeper understanding of love and grace. Accepting myself completely led to a fuller experience of peace and joy .

The red rubber ball I had bounced back when I was six-years-old has that lovely hollow twang once more. Each day is again filled with welcomed discoveries both fresh and sweet. My feelings are neither wrong nor right but just experienced.

——— *End* ———

Light in the Closet
TRANSGENDER SUPPORT

By providing relevant information, resources, practical help and emotional support, Light in the Closet hopes to:

1. Support the process of gender congruency.
2. Help individuals reconcile their faith, family obligations and transgender nature.
3. Encourage self-acceptance now, to help restore the individual's dignity and value.
4. Encourage personal growth and spiritual freedom through information and resources.

Most of us prefer to avoid the valleys. However, because Jesus promises to walk through the valley with us, the journey can be a fruitful one leading to godly growth.

Light in the Closet is here to help you understand your unique personhood and to shed light on your gender expression.

lightinthecloset.org

Light in the Closet

2800 Pleasant Hill Road, Suite 180

Pleasant Hill, CA 94523